Praise for
Narcissistic Abuse

"If you feel like you are treading water and cannot seem to find your footing, Vanessa M. Reiser provides hope, knowledge, validation, and a true clinical understanding so that you can become free from the vortex of cognitive dissonance and confusion that the narcissist purposefully spins you and entraps you in. She understands the family court system and ways to protect yourself. Her insights are authentic, well-studied, documented, and corroborated not just because she has experienced it herself but because she has made it her life's work to shine a light on pathological behaviors to help people not only recover but identify behaviors of abusers on a micro and macro scale so that future generations can also be insulated from dangerous people."

—Tina Swithin, author of *Divorcing a Narcissist*,
founder of One Mom's Battle, and advocate
for family court reform

"Vanessa M. Reiser's book on narcissistic abuse offers a truly unique perspective on the complex and often misunderstood topic of narcissistic mind control. By drawing parallels between narcissistic relationships and cult dynamics, the author provides readers with a fresh and intriguing lens through which to view manipulative behaviors and mind-control tactics. Vanessa's clinical understanding and groundbreaking insights make this book a must-have for your reading list."

—Dr. Nadine Macaluso, trauma bond and complex trauma
expert, psychotherapist, and author

"Vanessa M. Reiser is one of the most authentic, compassionate, and skilled clinicians I know in the mental health field. Her insights regarding narcissistic abuse and cult abuse are spot-on, not only because has she experienced it firsthand but because of the thousands of hours she's spend working with clients who have also experienced trauma at the hands of a narcissist/cult leader. She fuses the concepts of narcissistic abuse and cult abuse in a way that helps you deconstruct the concepts of mind control and manipulation in the most clarifying way."

—Debra Newell, *New York Times*
bestselling author of *Surviving Dirty John*

"Being in a narcissistic relationship can leave you feeling helpless, confused, isolated, and shameful. It can be extremely difficult to make sense of what is happening to you, making it difficult to leave. Vanessa M. Reiser breaks down these patterns in a comprehensive yet extremely empathetic way, making the reader feel seen without judgement. No matter where you may be in your healing journey, no matter what type of relationship you are in, Vanessa's book offers survivors compassion, direction, and a sense of empowerment to reclaim their sense of self."

—Dr. Jaime Zuckerman, licensed clinical
psychologist, author, and narcissistic abuse expert

"Vanessa M. Reiser's book is not only vital for anyone seeking to understand the dynamics of abuse endured, but ideally it ought to be required reading for young people—or anyone at all—so that this kind of abuse may be prevented. Vanessa's warmth and wisdom shine through in the way she breaks down this complicated subject in a useful and relatable way."

—Sarma Melngailis, author and businesswoman

Narcissistic Abuse

Narcissistic Abuse

A THERAPIST'S GUIDE TO IDENTIFYING,

ESCAPING, AND HEALING FROM TOXIC

AND MANIPULATIVE PEOPLE

VANESSA M. REISER, LCSW

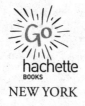

NEW YORK

Copyright © 2024 by Vanessa Reiser
Cover design by Amanda Kain
Jacket photograph by Des Panteva/Arcangel
Cover copyright © 2024 by Hachette Book Group, Inc.

Hachette Go, an imprint of Hachette Books
Hachette Book Group
1290 Avenue of the Americas
New York, NY 10104
HachetteGo.com
Facebook.com/HachetteGo
Instagram.com/HachetteGo

First Edition: October 2024

Published by Hachette Go, an imprint of Hachette Book Group, Inc.
The Hachette Go name and logo is a trademark of the Hachette Book Group.

The Hachette Speakers Bureau provides a wide range of authors for speaking events. To find out more, go to hachettespeakersbureau.com or email HachetteSpeakers@hbgusa.com.

Hachette Go books may be purchased in bulk for business, educational, or promotional use. For information, please contact your local bookseller or Hachette Book Group Special Markets Department at special.markets@hbgusa.com.

The publisher is not responsible for websites (or their content) that are not owned by the publisher.

Print book interior design by Bart Dawson.

Library of Congress Cataloging-in-Publication Data

Names: Reiser, Vanessa M., author.
Title: Narcissistic abuse: a therapist's guide to identifying, escaping, and healing from toxic and manipulative people / by Vanessa M. Reiser, LCSW.
Description: First edition. | New York, NY: Hachette Go, 2024. | Includes bibliographical references and index.
Identifiers: LCCN 2024031318 | ISBN 9780306833175 (trade paperback) | ISBN 9780306833182 (epub)
Subjects: LCSH: Narcissism. | Interpersonal conflict—Prevention.
Classification: LCC BF575.N35 R45 2024 | DDC 616.85/854—dc23/eng/20240709
LC record available at https://lccn.loc.gov/2024031318

ISBNs: 978-0-306-83317-5 (trade paperback), 978-0-306-83318-2 (ebook)

Printed in the United States of America

LSC-C

Printing 1, 2024

To my son, Anthony, who has always been my
greatest inspiration and teacher. Without his love,
I would not be the person I am today.

To all my clients, who are so courageous
and authentic in sharing their stories.

And to you, my readers: you are true warriors.

Out of suffering have emerged the strongest souls;
the most massive characters are seared with scars.

—

Khalil Gibran

Contents

Part III: Breaking Free

Author's Note

Stories here that are not my own are composites, with all names and identifying details changed to protect privacy.

Introduction
You Are Worthy

When I started to write the introduction to this book, I asked myself what made my story unique. Why would readers find my personal experience with a narcissist compelling or worthy? Out of the 158 million people in the US impacted by this insidious form of abuse, what makes me the right person to provide education to others about the red flags and warning signs they should look for?

Then, I remembered so much of the psychoeducation that I provide to my therapy clients when they are feeling disempowered. I encourage them to remember the things that they love about themselves, and so I am going to start by sharing with you what makes me uniquely positioned to offer advice and information on the subject of narcissism and narcissistic abuse. Although I have my flaws, as we all do, I'm really proud of my strengths. They have taken a lifetime to acquire and, believe me when I tell you, I did not take the easy road to get here, but now I can step back and honestly say that I am superstrong and have persevered through adversity in my childhood and my adult life.

I opened my own private therapy practice during the COVID-19 pandemic, and three years later, Tell A Therapist (tellatherapist.net) has five clinicians and support staff helping more than seven hundred clients.

While launching my business, I was actively working to overcome my own trauma as a victim of narcissistic abuse, ultimately running the equivalent of eleven marathons across the state of New York and then subsequently traversing across New Jersey, Connecticut, and Massachusetts in a wedding dress to raise awareness for this often misunderstood form of domestic violence. These experiences led me to this point, where I have developed mastery around something so difficult for so many to describe. It is my sincerest hope that the strength I have gathered over my own years recovering from narcissistic abuse translates into empowerment for you. I wanted to turn my pain into purpose, to give others a tangible road map to identify, escape, and heal from narcissistic abuse.

In preparation for this book, I used some of my own experience with various past relationships, collected stories from thousands of narcissistic abuse and cult abuse survivors, and sourced information from peer-reviewed articles, books, online forums, case studies, and my own friends and family. I have spent countless clinical hours helping people understand and heal from narcissistic abuse and relationship trauma. I share all these resources and experiences to create a comprehensive and therapeutically sound guide for your healing journey, because you deserve to feel validated, empowered, and refreshed in your heart and soul. You deserve to love yourself and be loved by others. Let's get started with unshackling you from the confusion and the potential notion that you are not worthy. You are more than worthy of peace and happiness!

WHAT IS NARCISSISM?

"Narcissism" is a popular buzzword that is frequently used to describe people that seem to love themselves excessively, have a big ego, or like to brag or take selfies. While the true narcissist may embody some or all of these characteristics, this is not what makes them so dangerous. The fuller definition of narcissism goes beyond the clinical and pop cultural ones, in insidious ways. In this book, I will explain exactly what a narcissist does that makes the psychological abuse they deliver so painful—and in some cases, fatal—for their victims.

Now, keep in mind that everyone is different, and abuse from a narcissist may be experienced differently, depending on one's relationship to the abuser. The way a child experiences their narcissistic parent may be different from how a partner experiences their romantic relationship with a narcissist. All victims of narcissists can certainly glean lessons from this book, but because of the focus of my clinical practice and my firsthand experience, this book's examples come primarily from romantic relationships with narcissists. That doesn't mean that they are not easily applied to a wide variety of relationships, because the narcissist's actions are predictable. Your narcissistic coworker may **love-bomb** you, so that you won't report them when you inevitably find out they've been skimming money off the top. A narcissistic neighbor many orchestrate a smear campaign about you around town, to discredit your version of events. They all follow the same playbook, and luckily, we can learn from it.

It is also important to point out that people who have been in a relationship or cult that included domestic violence, intimate partner violence, or **coercive control** (abuse hidden in plain sight) have gone through the same or similar experiences to those of survivors of narcissistic abuse. In fact, a romantic partnership with a true narcissist is what I like to call a "cult of one."

All cult leaders are either a narcissist, a sociopath (someone with antisocial personality disorder), a psychopath, or a person with overlapping characteristics from some or all of these, and they all use the same tactics that fall under the umbrella of brainwashing or mind control. Meanwhile, the progression of the relationship with a narcissistic partner, from the love-bombing early days that lure you in to the later and increasingly destructive cycle of wounding and soothing, mirrors the expectations of unfailing loyalty and constant attention that cult leaders as diverse as Jim Jones and Keith Raniere have sought from their followers. As such, I will use these terms interchangeably throughout this book, as well as the terms "victim" and "survivor," a nod to the fact that many individuals who have recovered from abuse have personal preferences as to which term should be used. I want to acknowledge and be respectful of both camps and certainly honor all of the stories of anyone victimized by a master manipulator.

MY STORY

I was born in New Rochelle, New York, the oldest of three children. My father was a telephone repairman, and my mother, an artist. My parents divorced when I was nine. I remember not hearing from my father for several months after he left, which was heartbreaking because I adored him. My grief was compounded by the fact that my mother was not always present.

My mother is a very talented artist. She gifted us with an understanding of the arts, music, and travel. She taught us how to take the nectar from the honeysuckle flower, and she was wildly free in her expression. We benefited tremendously from her ability to inspire us to become independent thinkers. My mother has also struggled with mania and depression for as long as I can remember. When she was depressed, she was not able to care for us adequately, and when she was manic, it was also hard. I sometimes felt like Cinderella, parenting my younger brothers and maintaining the home amid adverse conditions. I always wished that my mother would be more "like a normal mom," but she did her best.

When I was eighteen, my father died of cancer. I was devastated. So devastated that, in my twenties, I went to work for the phone company as a field technician, climbing poles just as he had. It created a connection between us that transcended his death and made me feel a little closer to him. I met my son's father at pole-climbing school, we got married, and I gave birth to our son. It was the first time in my life when I felt that I had a complete family. But relationships are hard work, and after eight years of marriage, his father and I called it quits. I still consider him a friend and a great co-parent.

After dating for a few years, I married someone who felt like the best friend and partner I had always been seeking. Around this time, I graduated from the University of Southern California at the age of forty-two, with a master's degree in social work and a focus on community organizing, which I put to use as a therapist at an outpatient triage-style mental health clinic as well as a social worker at a high school. This Irish ragamuffin had really turned her life around and found a way to turn pain into purpose.

I was blindsided when my second husband left me. I was shocked by the cruelty of his words when he told me with absolute indifference that he had never loved me. I thought I had found my lifelong companion, but his love turned off like a light switch, if indeed it had ever existed. Everyone thought we were the "perfect" couple. My reality shattered when the truth emerged. I didn't truly know the man I had shared my home, my bed, and my life with for all those years. It broke me. I was at a loss to understand how my life could've gone so off track. The pain was excruciating. Running was my solace. It seemed to get me grounded and reconnected to myself in the face of horrible realizations about my marriage and other things.

Then, I met the person who would love-bomb me by showering me with gifts and affection and then punish me to the extent that I would give up my sovereignty and my independence, so I would be easier to manipulate. This man came into my life when I was at my lowest point—by design—and he seemingly "fixed" everything with his beautiful words, loving demeanor, constant praise, and attentive nature. He was everything I could ever ask for. At the time, I was unable to take off the rose-colored glasses and realistically and critically consider his actions, words, intentions, and behaviors. I could not conceive that this seemingly genuine and authentic love was actually a fraud, a contrived tool to be wielded against me, used to control me.

Things moved quickly, as they do with a disordered person like this, and I ultimately fled the relationship. After I did, he threatened to ruin my life and destroy my social work license, and went on a smear campaign.

By this time, the **postseparation abuse** had begun, with one purpose: to keep me quiet about what I and the others before me had endured. Thankfully, I found a highly skilled attorney who was able to protect me. I alleged in court that my abuser even hired a private investigator to infiltrate my psychotherapy practice with fake clients posing as domestic violence victims. The family court did little to support me and berated me for "not looking like a victim." I believe this was because of all my advocacy work with my various runs across different states, and my being so outspoken on podcasts and other platforms. I work very hard to get the word out regarding narcissistic abuse in as many ways as I possibly can. It appeared as if the courts think victims are supposed to quietly hide under a rock somewhere. It was institutionalized "DARVO" at its best: deny, attack, and reverse the roles of victim and offender; it is supreme **gaslighting** when an institution claims you are responsible for what the narcissist is doing to you.

I began to learn everything I could about narcissism and found that all I had endured was in-line with what victims of narcissistic abuse experience. How had I not known about this? I was a therapist, but none of my training prepared me for what it would be like to live with someone who perpetually lashes out in anger, lies, manipulates, controls, isolates, punishes, threatens, intimidates, gaslights, and emotionally blackmails the person they supposedly love. If I didn't know about narcissistic abuse and I was a therapist, I was sure that so many others didn't know either.

After I fled my abuser, I came up with an idea. As a long-distance runner and two-time Ironman, I decided to combine my affinity for running with the need to shine a light on this worthy cause. I decided to run across the entire state of New York in a wedding dress to raise awareness of **narcissistic personality disorder (NPD)** and narcissistic abuse. I felt the dress was symbolic of the **future-faking** and fantastical thinking that the narcissist uses to exploit, control, and trap you. And on a personal level, retailoring my wedding dress served as an expression of me taking back my life, my inner essence: my sovereignty. I ran 285 miles across the state of New York, 55 miles across New Jersey, 60 miles across Connecticut, and 57 miles across Massachusetts, not just to be a voice for people, but also to remember the badass I was before this. It was transformative; it taught me you can be surviving and thriving at the same time.

It was a blessing to do that run and speak out for millions of silent victims. There have been so many gifts after this rebirth. I shifted my practice to focus on treating victims and survivors of coercive control, domestic violence, cults, and narcissistic abuse. I have learned that you can persevere and build a better life for yourself after narcissistic abuse, specifically because you sit in truth. **Truth is your antidote to the false world your abuser lives in.** You can begin to experience joy again and learn along the way who you are and have the happiness, confidence, and beauty that they never will. Step into your power.

—⟶∞⟵—

I want to be clear that this book isn't about me and what I endured, but my experiences do play a significant role in how I became an expert in the field of narcissistic abuse. This book is about YOU, the person seeking accredited information about this form of psychological and often physical abuse. If this book can change even one life for the better, open one person's eyes to what they are experiencing, I will have done what I set out to do. *Narcissistic Abuse* aims to shine a light on the trauma of narcissistic abuse, cult abuse, coercive control, and domestic violence. It is here as a resource to help those that have endured this trauma move forward in recovery. Throughout the coming chapters, I will share with you the lessons I have learned and the clinical background I have to help you heal. I will give you skills to help you break the **trauma bond**, and I will share exercises to help you become grounded. All will help you get into an empowered space and stay there.

You are powerful and strong. You have it within you. You always did. **I BELIEVE YOU.**

A QUICK NOTE ON HOW TO USE THIS BOOK

I wrote this with a particular trajectory in mind, tracing patterns that my clients and I have experienced, so the book may be most effective if you read it sequentially. That said, if certain chapters appeal to you more, go ahead and dip into those. I've included a glossary of common terms on pages 261–266, for easy reference; as already done in this introduction, the first text appearance of a glossary term has been bolded to alert you to its listing in the glossary.

While Chapter 17 is devoted to healing techniques, you will find a therapy tip at the end of every chapter. These tips aim to help you deal with some of the challenges that you may be facing at each phase of the book.

Some are evidenced-based practices and some are strategies that have added value to either my life or the lives of my clients. These are rooted in **cognitive behavioral therapy (CBT)** and **dialectical behavioral therapy (DBT)**. In simplest terms, cognitive behavioral therapy is a therapeutic practice that shifts cognition to a healthier inner dialogue; dialectical behavioral therapy includes very pragmatic approaches to emotional regulation.

Finally, but a very important content warning: I discuss in detail many types of abuse, including sexual abuse, perpetrated by narcissists against their victims. If, at any time, you are feeling activated, stop reading, practice some of the calming strategies on pages 110, and resume reading when you are ready. As I note later, you may also want to work with a professional therapist. You are a strong survivor and deserve all the external support you need and can get.

Part I

The Narcissist
You Love

To fully understand narcissistic abuse, you must first be willing to understand that people may have a different way of thinking than you do and that they may be eager to deliberately hurt others. I find that my clients' biggest barrier to processing and healing from narcissistic abuse is their trouble truly accepting this. Most people that struggle for the longest periods of time are stuck trying to apply logical thinking to the narcissist's behavior. They can spend decades spinning in the confusion because they are continuously applying a standard of thinking to the narcissist that is built on logic. The narcissist thinks *differently*! The narcissist does things to harm others for sport, and so you must unhand logic when you think about how they think.

The second thing that people really struggle with is the understanding that to remain around people like this is to have a loss of self. Many think that they can just fall in-line and they will somehow inspire the narcissist to behave like them or see things differently, but this is impossible, and the disappearing of self happens so slowly that you may not realize it until it is too late. There is no safe way to stay with a narcissist.

Chapter 1

The Most Important Thing: Your Safety

Like so many of my clients, when Kathleen first came to me, she was unsure what to call what she had been dealing with. For years, her husband (now ex) had manipulated her; she wasn't allowed to work outside the home nor did she have direct access to money (he said he was the man, he should provide, and he would give her what she needed). He also made sure that her kids were dependent on him, playing them against one another and her. He even tried to get an international divorce and continues to abuse her through the judicial system by filing thousands of motions against her for telling her story to others, managing to get her a sentencing. She is in her seventies and still cannot process what she has been going through. I shared the basics of narcissistic personality disorder with her; I let her know that narcissism and domestic violence go hand in hand. She realized that these rigid patterns are common with narcissistic abusers and their victims. This defining moment helped Kathleen understand what happened to her, name it, and start on the road of processing her trauma—and find true safety for herself.

3

———— ✺ ————

To ground us, I'll spend this chapter going over the basic elements of narcissistic personality disorder and then talk about what is the most important thing: your safety. While you may know some of this information, I encourage you to read through here, since it is critical to have a working knowledge of these signs and symptoms before we move on to other topics related to narcissistic abuse, including how to break free from the cycle.

I also want to take a moment to note that while you are reading, you might think, "Well, it's not that bad" or "He's nice . . . some of the time." When we live with and love a narcissist, we are trained to doubt ourselves and our experience. We are trained to gaslight ourselves! So, I ask you to trust yourself here as you read. I have been there and I am here for you. Knowing this information will help you protect yourself and keep yourself safe.

NARCISSISM 101

Narcissism is broadly defined as a fixation on oneself and one's physical appearance or the public perception of one's self. The *Diagnostic and Statistical Manual of Mental Disorders*, 5th edition (DSM-5),[1] describes narcissistic personality disorder (NPD) as possessing at least five of the following nine criteria:

- A grandiose sense of self-importance
- Preoccupation with fantasies of unlimited success, power, brilliance, beauty, or ideal love
- A belief that they are "special" and unique and can only be understood by, or should associate with, other special or high-status people or institutions
- A need for excessive admiration
- A sense of entitlement; unreasonable expectations of especially favorable treatment or automatic compliance with their expectations

- A state of being interpersonally exploitative (taking advantage of others to achieve their own ends)
- A lack of empathy (unwilling to recognize or identify with the feelings and needs of others)
- Envy for others or belief that others are envious of them
- Arrogant, haughty behaviors or attitudes

Two criteria of NPD that I want to underline here are the narcissist's need for excessive admiration and their lack of empathy. For the purposes of this book, all narcissists are, by definition, addicts because they are all addicted to attention and the dopamine kick they get from it. They will go to great lengths to find new victims, to give them a regular **supply**. What's more, lack of empathy shows how serious a condition NPD can be, as it is common ground in clinical portraits of narcissists, sociopaths, and psychopaths: without empathy, our humanity vanishes. Narcissistic personality disorder takes these two criteria and runs with them.

The original definition of narcissism and its current clinical identifiers do a disservice to the concept of narcissistic abuse, because it leads us to believe that this is a disorder in which the person loves themselves excessively. Not only does this not validate the severity of the trauma survivors of narcissistic abuse experience, which is similar to that experienced by victims of psychopaths and sociopaths, it also ignores a key component. The narcissist's baseline level of contentment is often lower than most other people's; in fact, narcissists will spend their lives trying to fill an inner void with sources of instant gratification, such as sex, food, drugs, porn, work, money, gambling, and video games, and they will crush anything that gets in their way. They may seem insatiable, and while there is no formal diagnosis of, say, food or sex addiction, there *is* an addiction to attention/dopamine. Without supply or attention, the narcissist decompensates; they feel hollowed out and will sulk or lash out, due to this overwhelming anguish. So, the narcissist's behaviors are not born of love, as in an earnest interest in their partner or offering emotional support; rather, they use the object of their affections as a temporary utility toward the goal of getting the next "fix," or drug. If you're not sure if you've been used for a fix, consider that narcissists may say things like "I just need five more minutes," if you're trying to get off the phone. They may even keep you on the line with them if you need to go to the bathroom, or they may need you to tag along when they're doing something that need not include you, such as going for coffee. They are not simply "in love with themselves," they hate being alone.

ORIGINS

There are many theories on where narcissism comes from, including a biological predisposition to NPD, childhood abuse, intergenerational trauma, or even social entitlement. According to the National Library of Medicine, the prevalence of lifetime NPD is 6.2 percent, with rates higher for men than for women (7.7% versus 4.8%).[2] According to narcissism expert Dr. Ramani Durvasula, approximately 1 in 6 adults is a narcissist that may or may not be diagnosed; I would posit that it impacts a higher rate of individuals overall.[3] This is because most narcissists do not get treatment; they see empathy as weakness or vulnerability, and they always need to feel that they are "winning." I also tend to lean toward there being a biological predisposition.

What makes the narcissist so hard to detect are the nuanced and subtle behaviors they exercise. Whereas *overt narcissists* may be terrifyingly and physically violent, as well as unabashed and unashamed of their selfishness in their pursuit of attention, *covert narcissists* have a sneakier approach and are better at keeping their "mask" on. The false self they present to the world is often so charming and so different from their true self that people fall prey to a vicious cycle that is extremely difficult to extricate themselves from. The victims of the covert or vulnerable narcissist stay longer and may end up with a lot more psychological damage because of the covert narcissist's finespun ability to cultivate doubts, inconspicuously manufacture insecurities, and gaslight. Many victims of narcissistic abuse don't even know for months or years that they are being abused, because of their narcissistic partner's covert nature.

Although the covert narcissist may originally mimic or copy their victim's interests and behaviors, utilizing a technique called **mirroring**, as well as shower them with gifts and praise—*love-bombing*—it is the narcissist's behaviors when the mask slips, such as being passive-aggressive, making demeaning statements, engaging in hot and cold behaviors, and blame-shifting, that chip away at the emotional strength of their victims. When their victims' emotional strength is depleted, they are better primed to supply the narcissist with admiration, praise, and whatever else the abuser may need. They become what Otto Fenichel calls a source of "narcissistic supply."[4]

THE ROLLER-COASTER RIDE

When you are in a relationship with a narcissist, you are on a roller-coaster ride of ups and downs that can also be called the *wound-and-soothe cycle*. This is because the **cognitive dissonance** that results from being in love with an emotional predator is enhanced by the false mask that the narcissist presents to the world versus who they are behind closed doors. Cognitive dissonance is the vacillation by the victim between their belief in the narcissist's false self and their realization of the narcissist's real self. In other words, it is the purgatorial state of having inconsistent thoughts, beliefs, or attitudes about your abuser. The narcissist may not always act like a monster, and the shifts between the two versions of them, the Dr. Jekyll and Mr. Hyde, create this dissonance. (Anyone who has to co-parent with a narcissist may have pretty serious cognitive dissonance, almost by design, because they have to believe the person that cares for their children will not harm them.)

Narcissists and cult leaders use similar tactics, such as the wound-and-soothe cycle, to enhance this dissonance and forge a severe *trauma bond*, which is when you find yourself addicted to the highs you experience when your toxic partner is trying to "fix" things. During this phase in the cycle of abuse, the toxic partner may look like they're trying to make up or do better; they may shower you with gifts again or pretend to be attentive to your needs. However, this makeup period is inevitably followed by a tension-building period, then a falling-out or a fight. This repeats over and over until you are ultimately discarded . . . or you leave.

This wound-and-sooth cycle is designed to confuse and control, even to the point of a victim not realizing they aren't their abuser's only source of attention.

IT'S NOT JUST YOU

Abusers will likely have a main supply of attention and admiration, along with other supplemental supplies. They may even call you by the wrong name or a nickname because they are not clear on who you are, other than someone to feed their needs, and they have too many people and lies that they are trying to remember. They will take attention from any person; their only deciding factor for a source of attention supply is "Does it have a pulse?"

Narcissists will use the same modus operandi (MO) over and over again to lure a new victim. They initially make contact under the guise of something benign, such as a business interaction or a coincidental "run-in." All of them turn happiness into sorrow, trust into disbelief, optimism into hopelessness, sovereignty into powerlessness, intelligence into dizziness, and open-mindedness into maladaptiveness.

BREAKING FREE

Once the abused person becomes aware of this cycle of abuse, they must practice self-care and detach with no contact with their abuser (or low contact if they have children together), or they will find themselves in a relationship of inevitable harm. This is because, when you give a narcissist what they want, they turn up the dial of abuse because they see that they can; if you do not give them what they want, they turn up the abuse dial because they feel entitled. You are damned if you do and damned if you don't. It's a losing game.

I would be remiss, though, if I didn't warn you that trying to detach from a narcissistic abuser is never easy. The narcissist will take good or bad attention as supply and will often be antagonistic to get supply from you, especially if they think you might leave. We will discuss more ways to get away later in the book, but it is generally the best idea to get away.

To sum up, and without mincing words, the narcissist is selfish, impulsive, dysregulated, boundaryless, and petulant; even though we know they are in pain and live in shame and darkness, they do little to work on themselves, so it is hard to have sympathy for them. They treat their supplies like an appliance or a toy that they will discard when it no longer serves them. They whimper and sulk because of their constant, unalterable hankering for the attention they're unable to give themselves, and if they don't get it, everyone around them will pay the price.

Many people don't understand narcissistic abuse: religious leaders, judges, therapists, friends, coworkers, attorneys, family members, and anyone who makes the mistake of saying things to you like "But he was nice to *me*" or "Why is it taking you so long to get over this?" or "But that's your mom" may be missing it. We are so sorely lacking in psychoeducation that victims are often not believed, furthering their victimization.

ALL DOMESTIC VIOLENCE IS NARCISSISTIC ABUSE

Narcissistic abuse is a specific type of domestic violence (also known as intimate partner violence) that is characterized by the creation of a false depiction of the abuser to gain access to and then take advantage of their victim(s). They create the false perception that they have their victim's best interests at heart when making decisions and in their behaviors initially feigning remorse for any "mistakes" or misdeeds. They then use a systematic and willful process of emotional abuse, psychological abuse and manipulation, financial abuse, and the myths believed in mainstream culture about domestic violence (e.g., it's only physical in nature or it only happens to people of a certain class) to gain and maintain power and control over their victim.

While not all perpetrators of narcissistic abuse would meet the criteria for NPD, they would likely rank very highly on a list of narcissistic traits. Just because it is hard to detect does not mean that this isn't domestic violence. It absolutely is. It is the trickery of it that makes it so sly, potent, savage, and soul-crushing.

All domestic violence is perpetrated through patterns of coercive and controlling behavior to maintain power within a relationship. Used by the narcissist, these acts are designed to make a person subordinate to and dependent upon their abuser by gradually isolating them from sources of support; exploiting their resources and capacities for personal gain; depriving them of the means needed for independence, resistance, and escape; and regulating their everyday behavior. Much of the work in this space targets violence against women within male/female intimate partner relationships, due to the quantifiable significance of this issue for women. Some abuse may be slower and less acute, but no less traumatizing. You could waste decades trying to deal with the confusion and cognitive dissonance that come with the narcissist's ever-changing personas.

As it currently stands, our clinical terminology comes up short when it involves discussions of "narcissistic domestic abuse." Because intimate partner violence indicates a relationship between partners, and domestic violence leaves out the clinical piece of narcissism, the term "narcissistic abuse" works to describe both the clinical piece *and* the domestic violence piece. I find that it is helpful for people to understand that psychological abuse is violent and that its falling-out is traumatic. Once you understand this truth, it is easier to see why all domestic violence is narcissistic abuse.

SAFETY

With all that foundational info in mind, I want to now address the most important part of our work: understanding safety. As the narcissist saps your energy (like a thought vampire or emotional cannibal) and manipulates you, they impact your well-being and your safety. Understanding how the narcissist operates is like a wake-up call. It will help you recognize these threats to your autonomy and agency, and it will prepare you for the work of distancing yourself from your abuser.

SELF-ACTUALIZATION AND THE NARCISSIST

When I first speak to someone who suspects they have endured narcissistic abuse, I always ask them, "Are you safe?"

A lot of my clients have been physically assaulted; many are also suffering from depression, anxiety, and extreme trauma responses to psychological and emotional abuse, which makes them vulnerable to a variety of safety issues, including suicide and homicide. While we honor your physical safety, your mental well-being is just as important. The damage done by psychological abuse is a trauma that you may not see outwardly but is entirely real and highly unsafe.

In clinical terms, Maslow's Hierarchy of Needs tells us that we need to be and feel safe before we can begin to focus on, much less do, much of anything else. Abraham Maslow first introduced his concept of a hierarchy of needs in his 1943 paper "A Theory of Human Motivation," in which he explained that people are motivated to fulfill basic needs before moving on to other more advanced needs. As a humanist, Maslow believed that people have an innate movement toward self-actualization, the realization of one's full potential. To achieve these ultimate goals, however, a number of more basic needs must be met, such as the need for food, shelter, and clothing. Maslow's hierarchy is most often displayed as a pyramid:[5]

The lowest levels of the pyramid are made up of the most basic needs (including the need for food, water, sleep, and clothing), while the most complex needs are at the top of the pyramid. Some of our basic safety and security needs including financial security, health and wellness, and safety against accidents and injury are almost always compromised when dealing with a narcissist.

Satisfying these lower-level needs is important to be able to avoid unpleasant feelings or consequences, but it is also necessary to progress to higher-level needs.

The next level includes things, such as love, acceptance, and belonging (e.g., friendships, romantic attachments, and social and community groups)—the emotional relationships that drive human behavior.

When the needs at the bottom three levels have been satisfied, our needs for esteem begin to play a more prominent role in motivating our

Maslow's Hierarchy of Needs

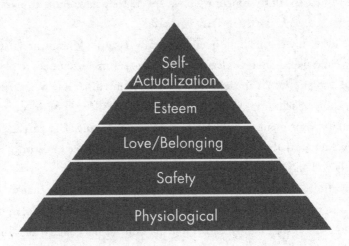

behavior as well as feelings of mastery takes priority. At this fourth level is the need for appreciation and respect.

At the very peak of Maslow's hierarchy are needs related to self-actualization. According to Maslow, self-actualization "may be loosely described as the full use and exploitation of talents, capabilities, potentialities, etc."[6] By definition, a relationship with a narcissist leaves you guessing; it will leave you unable to find safety, love/belonging, esteem, and let alone self-actualization.

A SCAN FOR SAFETY

With Maslow's hierarchy in mind, ask yourself these questions:
- How do you know you are/were in an unsafe place?
- Did you hear your gut or your intuition whispering things to you?
- Have you seen some red flags?
- What physical and emotional feelings did you have that gave you a warning? For example, did your heart beat faster or more frantically when your partner returned from work? Did you feel a clutching sensation in your throat?

If you answered yes to any of these questions:
- Did those negative sensations, thoughts, or emotional reactions distract your focus from things you enjoyed?
- Did they require you to go out of your way, taking up time and energy, to avoid experiencing them?

These indicators are your body telling you that you are not safe, much less able to focus on the higher-level needs that are important to you. Listen to them.

Chapter 2

The Narcissist's Calling Cards

It's a Monday morning and I have a new client. Ayla comes into session and is crying. She says she thinks she is married to a narcissist. I ask her why, and she shares that she caught him cheating and he is blaming her. He is also isolating her from her family and friends, and does not take any accountability. She starts asking me the standard questions, "Are they ALL the same?" "Why is he doing this to me?" "Can he change?" While I cannot diagnose someone that I have not met, I do share the checklist from page 4 because the list of common characteristics is a key component: it allows my clients to assess for themselves and make decisions accordingly.

———— ∞∞∞ ————

What can make pinpointing narcissism or NPD so hard are the nuanced and subtle behaviors narcissistic abusers may practice. It reminds me of the boiling frog analogy. If you plunge a frog into boiling water, it will immediately jump out, but if you place it into room-temperature water and slowly heat the water to boiling, the frog won't notice and will slowly cook to death. It's an apt analogy for how slow moving this trauma is.

This becomes even trickier to navigate when you consider that we all exhibit some level of narcissistic traits, though they're usually not indicators of clinical NPD. There are even healthy ways to be narcissistic—feeling proud of an accomplishment or celebrating yourself at an event, for example—but healthy narcissism is based in reality and on objective truths. There are low-range narcissists that are annoying with their various selfies on Instagram. There are midrange narcissists that are equal parts evildoer and martyr, and then there are malignant narcissists that are outright dangerous.

THE NARCISSISM SPECTRUM: FROM COVERT TO OVERT NPD

It's important to remember narcissism exists on a spectrum, and there are many different types of narcissism, with many people possessing some parts of *all* types. For the purpose of providing a clearer picture of the different kinds of narcissists, I'm going to stick with the basics and talk about the most common manifestations of NPD: overt and covert narcissism.

The Overt Narcissist

Also known as the *grandiose* or *malignant* narcissist, this person is assertive, extroverted, and a malicious emotional predator. This is the most severe subtype of narcissistic personality disorder. This person shows signs of sadism and aggression, and their narcissism may overlap with antisocial personality disorder/**sociopathy**. They are vindictive, antagonistic, and outwardly proud of their ability to get over on others. They have an unrealistic sense of superiority; an overestimation of their abilities; a propensity to dominate others; and an inflated sense of self-esteem, entitlement, braggadocio, and self-obsession. They enjoy seeing others hurt and confused, or both. These are the ultimate "one-uppers," who are highly competitive and will always need to win. Because an overt narcissist does not feel empathy, other people are merely a means to an end.

In spite of how awful these people sound, the overt narcissist is often able to surround themselves with admirers, due in part to their abilities to succeed in business or come off as someone of importance (sometimes faking academic success and entire careers with no credentialing). Overt narcissists choose professions that fulfill their need for power, attention, and superiority, such as surgeon, CEO, or actor. They are charming, smooth-talking, and likable while also being extremely jeopardous.

When it comes to the overt narcissist, superficial charm is a huge red flag. Because the overt narcissist often has a larger-than-life personality, people will tolerate abuse to be near them, especially because they are often wealthy, successful, seemingly important, and can offer relationship perks, but remember, the generosity of an overt narcissist is never without cost.

Despite their grandiose persona, the overt narcissist suffers from low self-esteem. They need positive affirmations, constant validation, and outright ass-kissing. They always have an agenda, and it is always self-serving. The overt narcissist is obsessed with their public persona, and often that persona includes being a great humanitarian. They are good at faking and can appear to be good listeners, generous, sensitive, loving, and faithful. However, all relationships are ultimately disposable to the ever-charming overt narcissist, and many victims suffer from mental, emotional, or psychological abuse at their hands. The overt narcissist will always demand their due, and if denied, they will often use whatever wealth and privilege they have to exact revenge. Additionally, if you look to expose them as the frauds they are or hurt their public persona, they will attempt to ostracize you from friends and family, potentially leveraging things of extreme value, such as your career or relationships, against you. Many narcissists are often misdiagnosed with bipolar disorder because the narcissist's grandiosity parallels mania in its symptoms of impulsivity, hypersexuality, and lack of sleep. Many will actually gladly accept this diagnosis to distract you from what is really going on.

The Covert Narcissist

The opposite end of the spectrum is the *covert,* or *vulnerable,* narcissist. As opposed to grandiose or overt narcissists, these people tend to be shy, self-effacing, inhibited, and modest. These may be poets, priests, or politicians. They try to hide their selfish manipulations and go incognito, with their condition undiagnosed. They often seem like the "guy/gal next door." The more overt narcissists seem to hit people over the head with their grandiosity and confidence, whereas the covert narcissist has a presentation of uncertainty and self-doubt. They may let other people make important choices for them because they say they feel indecisive and fear making a mistake; they will use such expressions as "I don't know" with a high level of frequency because they don't want to be responsible for any negative feedback.

All narcissists are quintessential cowards, but on the outside, a person with covert narcissism will seem quiet, meek, and self-deprecating. Instead of engaging with people, as does the overt narcissist, the covert narcissist will choose to be alone, not only because no one can live up to their high expectations, but also because they do not have the courage to endure any invalidating experiences. On the inside, though, despite all their jealousy, envy, overreaction to negative comments, and apparent shyness, the covert narcissist will feel, deep down, that they are better than other people. Because of their fluctuations between feeling superior and being jealous, and because they never feel satisfied or are able to form trust in others, the condition can result in despair, depression, self-injury, and even suicide.

WHY DON'T NARCISSISTS SEEK HELP?

Most narcissists do not really want to change. They are *ego-syntonic,* meaning they don't believe they have a problem. The disorder is consistent with their worldview, including their perception of others and perception of themselves.

If they do seek help, it is often because they are either mandated by the courts or convinced by their partners, or they do it to feel validated or to validate themselves to others. It's the "How bad can I be? I'm in therapy" game. There is also no real data that people with this disorder change, even when they seek help, because it is not possible to change their innate lack of empathy, which is ground zero for narcissistic personality disorder (more on this in Chapter 3). Any chance at a change would generally include long-term inpatient care, and their change would be measured in millimeters versus miles. It is also not recommended to go to couples' therapy with a narcissist because they glean information from the sessions and use it against you. Anytime you are in a relationship with a narcissist, it is one-sided, with them looking for all opportunities to exploit what they gather from you.

COMMON SIGNS AND SYMPTOMS OF NARCISSISTIC PERSONALITY DISORDER

If you suspect you've been or are being abused by a narcissist, you can use this guide to identify whether your experience puts you at a risk of violence, the draining of your energy or finances, or any other negative experiences you may have so you can escape. Keep in mind that all the characteristics of the narcissist are not well-documented in clinical books because they are very insidious and they are all working toward the goal of manipulating you. Manipulation is the overarching theme for them, and they are perpetually agenda driven with this in mind.

Again, I want to remind you that if you've been or are in a relationship with a narcissist, you have been gaslit—and love-bombed—and your own needs have been tamped down. Read about these signs and symptoms with an open mind; you may be aware of some, and you may have a terrible dawning realization about others. You may not have experienced all of these, and not every narcissist exhibits them all, but they are good for you to be aware of.

Addiction
Narcissists experience perpetual boredom, which is only made worse by an emotional shallowness, so they need to constantly seek ways to fill

that large void. They do this by finding external, temporary fixes. Narcissists are addicted to attention and the dopamine they get from it, but they also usually have addictions to drugs, alcohol, video games, work, gambling, food, sex, money, or porn.

LOOK FOR THIS: A partner who seems to be insatiable or perpetually unsatisfied. They seem to be unhappy in even the most ideal scenarios. They can ruin even the most amazing of things; they can never get enough sex, money, food, drugs (prescription or illegal), or attention. There is a "hole in the bucket," and they use a variety of addictive behaviors to try to fill this hole, to no avail.

Anxiety

Narcissists have no ability to regulate their own sense of self-worth, which is highly dependent on external feedback. This means that if something they say or do is ignored or their performance is given a lukewarm review, they are lost and puzzled, and their feelings of self-worth can be compromised, resulting in symptoms of anxiety. Keep in mind, many healthy people have anxiety, but narcissists tend to feel anxiety, perpetually, in part because of fear of exposure of their lies. Whereas the narcissist feels anxiety, the psychopath does not, and this may be important when identifying some of the characteristics that an abusive person in your life possesses.

LOOK FOR THIS: Someone who cuts lines, drives very fast, and paces around the house or yard. They may be a chain-smoker or have a hard time relaxing or sitting still. They also may not be good sleepers and may use or abuse sedatives or depressants to soothe their anxiety. Many will smoke cannabis to find relief. Many victims of narcissistic abuse report feeling the anxiety almost permeate their own skin, as if it were contagious; they enjoy when their narcissistic partner is high on marijuana because they get a reprieve from the punishment.

Being Boundaryless

When you are autonomous or expressing a need for privacy, the narcissist will push and challenge that and may slowly create a scenario in which you feel that you cannot do anything without your partner's permission, if at all.

LOOK FOR THIS: When you go to take a shower, they insist on pushing the door open to be in the bathroom with you, as a pattern of behavior, or will eavesdrop on your phone calls. They may even push past your secretary to gain access to you at work, or encroach upon your workspace in another way.

Braggart Storytelling

With their accounts of their amazing world and life, narcissists are hardly boring. The narcissist mesmerizes their audience with amazing facts, statistics, trivia and historical events, to the point that you feel overwhelmed and amazed by their acuity and accuracy. They are always the center of these stories, often rewriting their personal history and lying to embellish the stories. Think of Billy Joel's song "Big Shot," where the singer describes a boasting, blabbering, blowhard. They may tell you that they jumped out of a helicopter to go skiing with a famous person or that they have traveled to London over forty times, but they have never even been there. They may tell you that they graduated from Columbia Law School in convincing detail—they were so upset that their parents did not attend the graduation, but now they have been practicing law for many years—and yet they never attended law school.

The problem is, they pepper truths into their stories so as to create even more confusion. Narcissists work extremely hard at making themselves believable. They may also talk a lot and fancy themselves to be great conversationalists, but they are conversation hoarders; they may have a hard time ending conversations and will carry on far too long in their storytelling, braggart-style long-windedness.

LOOK FOR THIS: Someone who, when speaking, keeps you from getting a word in and monopolizes your time and attention. Someone whose stories don't add up or are riddled with inconsistencies and seem to be extreme exaggerations. They are very animated and can transfix a room of people with their circumferential theatrics. As they are engaging you in conversation, they expect eye contact and intense attention from the listener.

If the conversation strays to other subject matter, they tend to disengage incredibly quickly and visibly. You may notice this if you are in a social situation with them, at a party, or when they are telling you about their day.

Cheating

The narcissist cannot risk not having supply at any moment in time, so they generally have people waiting on the back burner to be ready if something is not going as planned with their main supply.

LOOK FOR THIS: Your partner has two phones or disappears for pockets of time, or you have a gut feeling that something is off. They generally have more than one intimate partner and will often visit with prostitutes—many of my clients are surprised to hear that they find the time, but they do!

Controlling

Every one of the characteristics listed here is designed to control you. That is the basis of manipulation by the narcissist to control your body, but moreover, your mind, so they can exploit you.

LOOK FOR THIS: The narcissist will demand to know who you see and who you talk to. Many will even take over your phone or email address as well as your social media accounts. They may control what you eat and when, what you wear, and where you go. This may manifest in their monopolizing all your time and managing your appointments, with punishment if you do not follow their ways.

Deflection

When you are communicating with a narcissist, you may notice that they have a hard time answering a direct question. They may sidestep questions and be evasive. This can be because they may be trying to buy time to gather up a good lie in their mind or they want you to continue to query them as a way to get attention from you. When someone lies as much as they do, it can become customary to have so many lies circulating that they have to constantly cover their tracks.

LOOK FOR THIS: Someone who cannot commit to an answer, answers a question with another question, or is perpetually defensive.

Some may change the subject or tell you "that was in the past" as a way to get off the topic and deflect away from their bad behavior or desire to cover up a lie. It is a form of gaslighting because you may find yourself extremely confused when you get into communication patterns like these.

Entitlement

The narcissist may come off as grandiose and seek to get ahead of others because they feel entitled to "win" and they may treat the world as their playground.

LOOK FOR THIS: They cut lines, drive fast, and seem to want to one-up everyone around them and win at all costs. They may also feel entitled to your time, sex, money, or attention.

Fantastical or Magical Thinking

For the narcissist, *fantastical* or *magical thinking* is different from a New Age belief in the power of the will or the law of attraction. The narcissist believes that they can influence the world around them with their thoughts, that just their thinking makes it so because they have some inner magic that others do not have. This is something we see in children who believe wholeheartedly that if they wish for something, they will get it.

Narcissists never grow out of this belief. They often become frustrated, angry, and upset if more is required of them—such as actual work. They believe they need only manifest things and some magical force will make it so. (Oddly enough, it *does* work for them a lot of the time, in a manner of speaking. Sometimes, **flying monkeys**—enablers—step in and rescue narcissists from the consequences of their own bad decisions, and this becomes proof to the narcissist that their magical thinking is correct.)

Whenever things don't go the narcissist's way, any cracks in their delusion will cause them to become irritated or even rageful. The narcissist does not do well with any realistic conversations, so if you have an illness or have a sick family member, the narcissist may even see your illness as a weakness in your character. Put simply, they are allergic to reality.

LOOK FOR THIS: Some examples of magical thinking might be "I can drive as fast as I want. Other cars will get out of the way," or "I never get sick." You may spend hours arguing, explaining, and trying to convince the narcissist that the way they are behaving is dangerous, unfair, and irresponsible. When you or someone you love becomes ill or injured, the narcissist will not be able to show up in the way that someone who truly loves you would. They will see your illness or injury as a threat to their perfect fantasy life. Additionally, if you question their magical thinking, you will be accused of trying to cause problems or derail their plans. They may tell you that they "manifested" your coming into their life. They may sell you on "the story" of your meeting and feel angered by your not subscribing to "the fairytale story" as if the universe had somehow played a role in your colliding by magically putting you in front of each other and it was "meant to be." More than likely, you were stalked and preyed upon.

Future-Faking

The narcissist also future-fakes: makes promises with no intention of fulfilling those promises. They might facilitate the bonding and connection in a romantic relationship by promising to pay for your education, buy you a car, or give you a family, but never quite deliver. Even when they "buy" you a car, they may make a down payment, but then saddle you with the monthly expenses. The narcissist will give you a kidney on Monday and discard you on Tuesday. In other words, they confuse you by sometimes coming through on promises, but mostly they are not delivering on them. It's a con job. Future-faking convinces you to stick around because the stakes get higher and higher.

LOOK FOR THIS: A person telling you that they will buy you a house, give you a leg up in your career, or provide you with the family you have always wanted. They peddle a fantasy, but beware of someone wanting to get on your mortgage or the deed to your house, or wanting to open a mutual bank account early in the relationship. These grand promises of a blissful future sound great, but the narcissist will keep moving the goalpost and inevitably disappoint you. As the relationship grows and the narcissistic partner begins to lose interest, the gifts and kind gestures will fade, but if you begin to pull away, question things, or try to slow down the trajectory, the narcissistic partner will show disapproval or become dismissive.

Gaslighting

Gaslighting is a hallmark of narcissists and narcissism. It is a form of psychological manipulation in which the abuser attempts to sow self-doubt and confusion in your mind. Typically, gaslighters distort reality and force you to question your own judgment and intuition. The term "gaslighting" comes from the 1938 play *Gas Light*, which George Cukor adapted into the 1944 film *Gaslight*, in which a man tries to convince his wife that she is going insane; gradually she begins to question her own memories and perceptions.

Gaslighting can look like circular conversations in which the narcissist seems to use a jumble of incoherent speech, called "word salad," or keeps talking about the same issue over and over again. It can be blame shifting, whereby they blame you for their bad behavior, or they may even take you down a different road when you ask a direct question. They might spend hours "talking in circles" with you and may even get physically aroused while arguing. An abuser may accuse you of "turning them off" when you defend yourself and argue or become reactive with them. This is a lie. They enjoy it and are turned on by it. You may sometimes feel stupider after these lengthy conversations.

After being gaslit, many people develop stuttering, confusion, problems focusing, and depression, among other symptoms. Others report having a hard time trusting themselves, trusting others, or making even the simplest decisions. They begin to second-guess themselves, walk on eggshells, and believe they are incapable or "less than."

Live in your truth. You are not imagining things. If it happened, it happened. The truth doesn't change even if the narcissist in your life says so or a zillion of their friends agree. There are no such things as "alternative facts."

LOOK FOR THIS: The gaslighting narcissist will use *mirror statements* like a snake oil salesman. This is when they take the last word of the sentence you just said and use it to flip the entire narrative, stealing your perspective. It may look something like this:

Victim: "I can't believe you are doing this again. I can't breathe."
Narcissist: "Breathe? I can't breathe."

In this common scenario, the narcissist robs you of your perspective and steals your narrative, which is designed to break you down and get you to react.

Another good example is when they minimize their hurtful behaviors or words by saying something like "It was just a joke" or "You're way too sensitive." Anytime you are made to feel crazy or question the truth in a conversation, you may be getting gaslit. More nuanced behaviors may be anytime a narcissist sidesteps a question or doesn't answer the question. The bottom line: gaslighting is designed to confuse you. Beware the circular conversations, sidesteppers, and question evaders. Another, more insidious form of gaslighting includes moving your belongings around so that you begin to think you are going crazy, or cybergaslighting, when they hack into your iCloud or do something using technology to have you question reality.

Impulsivity

Narcissists may say and do things that offer short-term or even immediate gratification over long-term benefits. They may think they are impervious to repercussions or consequences, especially as they relate to the law. They are impulsive because they have enthroned their primal animalistic urges—fear, jealousy, anger, lust—the way a small child would.

The narcissist worships their impulsive urges and follows them as much as they can because they think they are right, good, and correct. If they are jealous, then they are right to be jealous, and they are right to do whatever their jealousy tells them to do to soothe themselves.

LOOK FOR THIS: An unwillingness to practice safe sex, driving recklessly, not obeying the law, booking elaborate trips to commence the next day, bingeing, making large purchases, changing automobiles with a high level of frequency, moving frequently, or being unaffected by the prospect of repercussions or consequences. If they are a parent, they will leave their children unsupervised to do whatever makes them happy in the moment. The real problem with impulsivity is the proclivity to act upon sometimes dangerous urges to harm others.

Insecurity

Narcissists use "compensatory adaptation to overcome and cover up low self-worth," according to a psychology paper published in 2021 in the journal *Personality and Individual Differences.*[1] Narcissists cope with their insecurities by this "flexing." You may also notice that they have few or no friends that are not business associates; they may avoid group activities or have little to no hobbies of their own. Anytime the focus is not on them, they may become triggered.

LOOK FOR THIS: So many victims report that the narcissist ruins birthdays and holidays, and this is because they need to be the focus of everyone's attention. The special occasions take the focus off them and put it onto others, thereby infuriating the narcissist because of their high levels of insecurity. We sometimes refer to the holiday season (October to January) as "narc [narcissist] season," because of their challenges. Another indicator is when they have to put others down to feel better about themselves. If you excel in your career or any facet of your life, the narcissist is sure to become triggered.

Intimidation

Whether it is physical, verbal, or mental, the narcissist uses intimidation so that you'll fear them, thereby conforming to their demands. Early on, they may reprimand others in front of you so as to plant the seeds in your mind that, if you mess with them, you, too, will receive their wrath. They also use intimidation to manipulate you and cause more confusion within your own mind, with subtle threats that make you wonder whether it's real or they're messing around. They do this on purpose so that, while you are worried about the threat, you don't want to make a fuss.

Intimidation can be a form of gaslighting. After all, you might fear that if you speak out or say something to other people, they won't believe you. They might think you're overreacting, as the narcissist will tell you and others, "You're too sensitive," "You're overreacting," "You are imagining things," or "Everyone thinks you are wrong." You are not overreacting; all threats should be taken seriously.

LOOK FOR THIS: Intimidation can take many forms; it can be as overt as physical assault (hair-pulling, pinching, biting, force-feeding you, forcing you to have sex, or strangling you to make you scared but maybe not enough to leave). The narcissist may block you from leaving a room, padlock you out of the house, shut down credit cards or bank accounts, scream at you when you are trapped in a moving vehicle, take your phone, or threaten you with statements like "You'll never see the children again" or "I am going to ruin your career." They may do things like get in your face, break things, or punch walls; they may destroy your property (e.g., by bleaching or cutting clothing or other belongings), raise their voice, hide passports, or share with others a secret that they know about you. Some may even text you threats from phantom numbers or drive by your home, and make you start to live in fear. They may record you in or out of the home and blackmail you with any of the data that they have recorded. Some may fake phone calls or have real-life negative engagements with subordinates, yelling directives at them, so that you overhear it and become nervous or fearful. They may clean their firearms in front of you or flex with waitstaff in a way that shows they are in charge, as a way for their victims to be nervous and afraid of them. Whether overt or covert, the narcissist will always find a way to justify their behavior because it is designed to gain a level of tolerance to the abuse, and it will always escalate. Any threat should be taken seriously. You are not imagining or exaggerating things.

Isolation

One of the biggest tools that the narcissist uses is to remove any support systems that you may have. They will slowly bad-mouth your friends and family to get you to move away from your support system and rely more and more on them, and only them, over time.

LOOK FOR THIS: Distance and time between you and the people that you love. The narcissist will plant seeds about your family, friends, and colleagues, and the way that they treat you to try to put wedges between you. They might also take you on trips, occupy your energy, or complain that you are spending too much time with others—all so much that you have very little time to devote to the relationships that are historically yours. In a marriage, they may move you out of the state or region that you live in.

Love-Bombing

You may notice early on that the narcissist is fast-moving. You may move in together after a very short period of time. They may say that they love you soon after meeting you or refer to you as their "soulmate" at an extremely early stage in the relationship. You may become engaged quickly, or they may ask you to elope early on. In this love-bombing phase, they are calling constantly, and their texts are incredibly long and emotive. They're always giving you compliments, and they want to meet your parents or introduce you to theirs, even though you've been on only a handful of dates.

To be clear, not everyone who is affectionate and overeager is someone with NPD. The devaluing phase is actually what makes you learn that it was love-bombing, and we will talk more about that later. Their efforts early on are to get you addicted to them as they are addicted to your attention.

LOOK FOR THIS: The narcissist will send lengthy text messages, going on and on about how you are their soulmate and you are meant to be together. They profess that they've never felt this way before and that fate played a role in getting you together. There will be a vibe about the relationship that feels "too good to be true." They will lavish you with compliments, cash, jewelry, tickets to concerts, trips, cars, houses, puppies, long poems, flowers, love notes, texts, calls, surprise visits, and generally over-the-top positive experiences, leading you to feel intoxicated, yet unbalanced and eventually fatigued.

Lying

Narcissists lie, exaggerate, and confabulate, or fill in the blanks when they forget the truth. They are oftentimes deluded and may even believe the lies they are spewing about themselves or others. Remember: They have been at this for their entire lives, so they become good at bullshitting. Many narcissists will even tell you such things as they have traveled to various countries they have never visited, or they were an executive at a company where they never worked. Their narratives support their fantastical thinking and they have a limitless ability to self-enhance and amplify their personas, due to the internal void they long to fill.

LOOK FOR THIS: Their lips are moving. Actually, their lips do not need to be moving, because they often believe their own bullshit. The narcissist is living a lie, and it is so pervasive that it may be hard to detect. Don't let them gloss over inconsistencies, and do not make excuses for those inconsistencies. The benefit of the doubt is the narcissist's best friend. Do not give anyone "the benefit of the doubt." Fact-check, listen to your gut, and keep a log so that you can see whether patterns develop. There are many overlaps between lying and gaslighting, such as when you catch them in a lie but they convince you of something else. They will sometimes also omit information, so keep fact finding.

Mirroring

Narcissists live vicariously through you. By mirroring your personality quirks, as well as your likes and dislikes, they are trying to give you what you want as a way to win you over. While they lack a strong sense of self, one strength narcissists do have is the ability to watch others closely and then use this information in their favor to mimic it. A narcissist seems to always know what you like, and then give that to you. It feels as if they know you so well and are invested in your happiness. When they can provide you with something you like, they can win you over and better control and manipulate you. This mirroring is the most prominent during the love-bombing stage. Mirroring is a way to keep control of the relationship while increasing the chances their partner will stay and continue to serve as the narcissistic supply they need. During the initial stages of a relationship, mirroring can be flattering. This person appears to be behaving in a way that suggests they listen to you and care about the same things you do, even adopting your political views, taste in automobiles, interior decorating, music library, cultural interests, and so on. This causes problems for people when they ultimately get away because they have been mirrored so much that they think they are the narcissist. One way to discern this is to see who the *proactive* person is, and who, the *reactive* person. The narcissist is the proactive person because they are always working with an agenda and the victim reacts.

LOOK FOR THIS: They adopt your hobbies, culture, music, and even wear clothing that you like. If you are a triathlete, they will buy a bike, even if they cannot ride, and start to practice. If you are Italian, they will start to call you by an Italian name or nickname and learn what they can about that culture to make you think they care about it or you. Beware of the person who makes your favorite song their ringtone or starts to behave like you and yours.

No Empathy

There is an entire chapter devoted to this, but it is important to add it to the playbook. The nature of the narcissist's disorder affects their ability to feel emotional empathy. It is extremely diminished.

LOOK FOR THIS: A partner or family member who does not care whether you, your children, your family members, or your pets are sick. The narcissist may even accuse people of deserving their illnesses or blame them for it, or claim that nothing is really wrong with them, shaming them.

Passive Aggression

Passive aggression is a way of expressing negative feelings, such as anger or annoyance, indirectly instead of directly. Because the narcissist is not insightful and a terrible communicator, they will be snarky and snide and give jabs when they are punishing you.

LOOK FOR THIS: They will say things with a happy voice, but you know they are lying. Many narcissists will use this as their primary dialogue, saying untruths that are tied in a bow. If you ask them a question, they may respond condescendingly or patronizingly or be sarcastic or snarky in their communications with you.

Projection

Projection is easily confused with mirroring, but the two things are distinctly different. *Mirroring* is reflecting an image back. *Projecting* is casting an image as if onto a blank screen. In psychological terms, projections can be positive or negative, but they are always external representations that may bear little to no relationship with the person they are ascribed to. Narcissists project their own traits, actions, values, fears, fantasies, desires, hates, motives, and distorted self-beliefs onto others. People with NPD habitually scapegoat negative traits onto those around them. The cerebral cortex has also been found to be less developed in narcissists, and this area of the brain is responsible for memory, emotions, and behavior.[2] Therefore, the narcissist seems to move on so fast because their emotions are not as deep as ours, nor do they form memories or have sentimentality, nostalgia, or attachments in the same way that the rest of us do.

LOOK FOR THIS: The narcissist's accusations are confessions. If they tell you that you are a cheater, they are cheating. They literally tell you who they are and what they are doing! If the narcissist is accusing you of something that you *know* you didn't do, they are giving you intel into what they are doing. If they tell you that you are going to go to prison, they are telling you that they are engaging in criminal activity.

Silent Treatment

This is when the narcissist ignores you to punish you, as a way to manipulate you into chasing them or falling in line with something they want from you.

LOOK FOR THIS: Your partner hides in a different room in the house, stops responding to messages or calls, disappears for pockets of time, or refuses to engage with you at all.

Smear Campaign

This is one of the phases in the cycle of abuse, so we'll talk more about this in Chapter 12, but in short: A **smear campaign** begins while the narcissist is still with you, but it comes out in the open and goes full force once the relationship with the narcissist is devolving, after the "discard," or the breakup (Chapter 11). It is a form of damage control used by narcissists when they become aware that they have been exposed. Smear campaigns are frequently used to depict the victim as insane, bipolar, having borderline personality disorder, having Munchausen syndrome by proxy, an addict, alcoholic, unstable, a gold digger, thief, cheater, or poor parent.

LOOK FOR THIS: The charming ability of most narcissists is remarkable as they easily transform from an angry monster inside the house to perfect neighbor outside. This flawless performance is the ideal groundwork to emphasize their victim's overreactions and smear them. They will claim their spouse is crazy by citing some visible tantrums while minimizing their contribution to those tantrums, but nothing compares to the pageantry of the narcissist in court. They are vexatious litigants and will file excessive lawsuits designed to intimidate and scare their spouse into submission.

Superficiality

The narcissist is oftentimes emotionally unintelligent, shallow, and superficial, coveting things that are unimportant or visual, such as fancy cars, watches, and homes. Because someone with NPD lives in a fantasy world, they will want things that make them appear to be financially successful, even if they are not.

LOOK FOR THIS: Someone who seems to be too excited by famous people, likes on social media, or other items that are not sentimental or add intrinsic value to your life. They may prefer to rent a house for far above their budget in an area that is desirable just so they can say they live in that area, even if they are throwing their money away in rent. Some may even be homeless but still have a Rolex or boat. For them, it's all about the optics.

Transactional Relationships

Narcissists have no real friends, only business dealings. You are one of their business dealings. *Anything* they do for you is done so that you will have to pay them back in some way. If the narcissist buys you something or does anything for you, get ready for them to ask for something in return, and if you do not supply it, get ready for the rage, silent treatment, or other punishment. They want kudos for simply getting the mail, taking the dog for a walk, fixing the leaky sink, scooping the kitty litter, or taking your car for an oil change, and a simple "Thank you, babe" will not do. They want extreme worship and dramatic public praise or else, but keep in mind that you can never live up to their expectations. They set you up to fail, because even if you do what they want, they will turn up the dial and deliver more devaluing.

It is not just material things you might owe the narcissist, but sex and services. You are just a tool for them, so even though they pretended to be interested in you in the beginning, ultimately, they will reveal that they entered the relationship as a user. You're as personal to them as an interaction with a grocery store cashier, which is to say, barely at all.

LOOK FOR THIS: They use salutations or transactional language but at odd times, such as the inappropriate use of "I'm sorry" or "thank you." They may thank you for something that you imagined was mutually enjoyed, like sex or a peck on the lips, which is an indication that they were using you. They may also apologize after sex, indicating the same. They also have a hard time receiving gifts because they think you are trying to manipulate them.

Triangulation

Narcissists may pull a third person into your relationship to create conflict between you both so they can better manipulate and take advantage of you by cultivating an insecurity in you. This is **triangulation**.

They may play the role of messenger between you and another person, making sure that there is limited or no communication between the two of you, except through the narcissist. They do this to invoke feelings of insecurity and jealousy—also to maintain control in the relationship. For example, they might tell you about a coworker or friend who keeps flirting with them, creating an illusion that they are desirable. This may cause you to feel insecure and afraid that your partner may leave you. They may alternatively tell you stories of how their ex treated them poorly to summon feelings of loyalty and get all your attention. They usually create a narrative that their exes are all "crazy" because they not only actually believe this, but they do not want the new supply to communicate with the exes and find out the atrocities they have committed. Narcissistic parents often create conflict between their children as a way to triangulate.

LOOK FOR THIS: A partner who tries to bring their children, friends, family, neighbors, or business associates into arguments to bolster their angle. They may turn to a cohort or flying monkey (enabler) and say, "Right, Jane?" Pay attention to the "faces of narcissism" on the flying monkeys or other people (family members, business associates, and former victims) around the narcissist. Some people may look fearful. Some may look concerned. Some may be unaware. Some may wear their concern, confusion, or their "here we go again" perspective on their face.

Wearing a Mask

Whereas overt narcissists may be terrifyingly and physically violent, as well as unabashed and unashamed of their selfish pursuit of attention, covert narcissists have a sneakier approach and are better at keeping their "mask" on. The false self they present to the world is often so charming and so different from their true self that people fall prey to a vicious cycle that is extremely difficult to extricate themselves from. The covert narcissist has a finespun ability to cultivate doubts, inconspicuously manufacture insecurities, and gaslight, all while seeming to be a loving partner. You may not realize you are a victim of narcissistic abuse for months, years, or even decades because of your narcissistic partner's covert nature. The more covert narcissist might portray themselves to the public as a philanthropic and kind soul while behaving alternatively vindictive and retaliatory behind closed doors.

LOOK FOR THIS: A high contrast between what the narcissist looks like in public and how they behave when not many people can see them is a hallmark of narcissism. They often portray themselves to the outside world as an overly dedicated parent, lovesick Romeo, poor victim, charismatic leader, generous philanthropist, heroic martyr, expert on everything, loyal friend, or highbrow intellectual. They may make large donations to community organizations while being dark and solemn in private.

Withholding

Narcissists deliberately hold back an emotional reaction or connection and get a thrill when they leave you wanting more. The narcissist will make a point of **withholding** something that they know you really want or need as a form of control.

Another, more insidious tactic they use is the harboring of valuable information or items to maintain control over you. If they detect that you have attached a value to something, it becomes valuable to them so they ultimately destroy it or keep it from you. Many of my clients report things they considered precious went missing or were used to blackmail them, including sensitive information or intimate photographs.

LOOK FOR THIS: Withholding can manifest itself in someone who is deliberately late, gives you the silent treatment, or gives you only breadcrumbs of love. You may sometimes see this in brief conversations in which you simply ask a narcissist how their day was, and they answer with a mere "I don't know," thereby punishing you by withholding information and making you feel that you are not deserving of this information and connection.

Wounding/Soothing

As introduced earlier, the *wound-and-soothe cycle* is a repetitive string of hot and cold behaviors that narcissists engage in. After the initial love-bombing phase of the relationship, as the narcissist needs more and varied forms of attention from their supply, they might be passive-aggressive (or downright aggressive); might get upset, pick fights, and use the silent treatment or the disappearing act; then apologize and start love-bombing again. It is a confusing roller-coaster ride, with victims left clinging to occasional scraps of affection. It begins to break you down, and you start to lose your sense of self.

This cycle only prolongs the inevitable and causes you to stay in toxic relationships for far longer than is healthy for you. In the end, the inevitable will happen, but it becomes increasingly difficult to remove yourself from this cycle, and then the journey to recovery is very long and difficult.

LOOK FOR THIS: A narcissist will purposely cause a fight before a big party and then, at the last minute, make up with you to seem like the hero that sacrifices their own feelings to make you feel better. They may even secretly cancel a flight, then be the hero that fixes the issue and gets you on the next flight. They will cause a problem and then fix the problem.

—❦—

There's a lot of information to digest here and you may be feeling activated; here are some quick things to do that can be helpful in getting you emotionally regulated after dealing with some of the traumatic events that you may have experienced or are experiencing.

THERAPY TIP: EMOTIONAL REGULATION

Some dialectical behavioral therapy (DBT)–based skills that may help include:

- Taking a walk, whether alone or with a loved one
- Journaling about what you're feeling
- Practice box-breathing:

Step 1: Breathe in, slowly counting to four.

Step 2: Feel the air enter your lungs. Hold your breath for 4 seconds. Try to avoid inhaling or exhaling for 4 seconds.

Step 3: Slowly exhale through your mouth for 4 seconds.

Repeat steps 1 through 3 until you feel re-centered.

- Do a body scan:

Pay attention to all parts of your body and bodily sensations in a gradual sequence from your feet to your head.

Step 1: Get into a comfortable position, either lying or sitting down.

Step 2: Close your eyes.

Step 3: Deepen the breath and bring awareness to your body.

Step 4: When ready, breathe in and bring awareness to either your head or your toes.

Step 5: Notice and pay attention to any sensations, such as tingling, tightness, or discomfort.

Step 6: After scanning one part of your body, move on to an adjacent part. For example, if starting at your head, move on to the neck, then the shoulders, then your chest, and so on. Continue in this way along your entire body.

Step 7: Once the body scan is complete, get up slowly.

Chapter 3

Empathy Not Included

When I first gave birth to my son, I really had no idea what I was doing. I was pretty young and didn't have any gauge or frame of reference for what motherhood would entail. Even though I had read books on parenting, nothing would truly prepare me for this incredible experience. I had never experienced a love like this, and I quickly discovered that I would be intensely interested in meeting this child's needs. When this new cherub would start to cry, I innately found a way to soothe him, whether it was through a feeding, changing a diaper, or rocking him to sleep. If I had noticed that he was upset but hadn't felt intensely emotional about helping him stop crying, I may not have been as motivated to drop everything and help him. Without my care, he would have become damaged or even died.

Empathy is what keeps our species going. Without it, we are doomed.

When I was mothering my baby, I didn't really think about em-
pathy so specifically; it came naturally to me—it was just what I did.
But when I was in a relationship with a narcissist and in the trauma
work I did after, I realized that a lack of empathy is one of the biggest
calling cards of a narcissist.

⚬⚬⚬

A lack of empathy is ground zero for narcissists; it warrants its very own chapter, as it is the key factor found in all narcissists and it accounts for so much of their malignant behavior. Although this may be difficult to read, understanding this and other elements of "Narcissism 101" will help you gain perspective on the actions and behaviors of the narcissist in your life.

WHY DO NARCISSISTS LACK EMPATHY?

When you buy a new electronic toy for a child, the packaging often says, "Batteries not included." Similarly, the narcissist should come with a warning label that reads, "Empathy not included."

According to the *Diagnostic and Statistical Manual of Mental Disorders*,[1] narcissists are "unwilling to recognize or identify with the feelings and needs of others." Research shows, though, that this lack of empathy goes beyond being "unwilling" to feel for other people.[2] Narcissists have structural abnormalities in brain regions associated with empathy. Hence, their ability to appropriately respond emotionally and to express care and concern for others is significantly impaired.

It is critical to remember that narcissists are indifferent to your pain, suffering, or sadness. They might *fake* empathy—portraying themselves in a certain way and playing the game—but only so that they can get their own needs met.

WHY IS A LACK OF EMPATHY SO DAMAGING?

For someone to be empathetic, they must be able to recognize and understand other people's emotions (*cognitive empathy*) and to *feel* them (*affective empathy*). For example, when someone with empathy sees someone else in distress, the empathetic person instantly recognizes and understands that the person is sad or in pain, and at the same time, they start to feel sad or pained themselves. They have the ability to put themselves in someone else's shoes. Together, cognitive empathy and affective empathy give rise to the overall experience of empathy; thus, intact functioning of both is necessary for optimal empathic response. A long history of theory and research indicates that empathy plays a key role in morality, prosocial behavior, and inhibiting antisocial behavior.

Put simply, empathy is the fundamental basis of our existence.

EMPATHY AND THE BRAIN

Narcissistic individuals have *both* lower cognitive *and* affective empathy. The data also suggests that narcissists perform better when it comes to cognitive empathy but not affective empathy, indicating that they can fake, in a variety of ways, emotions they recognize in others, such as faking crying.

For example, when asked to look at pictures of people's faces or to watch video clips showing other people expressing various emotions, narcissistic individuals are able to identify each emotion as well as less narcissistic people do, but they report feeling the emotion shown on-screen to a lesser extent as compared to a less narcissistic person.[3] It is likely that being able to understand others' emotions—but not feel them—is one of the mechanisms by which narcissistic individuals are able to treat others in such a callous manner.

This may also help explain why they struggle to remember people and faces. In a study conducted in 2021, narcissists were found to exhibit poor recognition memory; this is thought to come from an excessive self-focus and from the tendency to disregard the needs of others. This leads them to have a hard time recognizing people, remembering names, drawing faces, and forgetting details about their surrounding environment.[4]

CAN THE NARCISSIST BE "IN LOVE"?

In a word, no. A narcissist may *possibly* care for anyone in a moment that is serving their purposes, but that is it.

Narcissists have a few hurdles to genuinely loving another person. First, they see neither themselves nor others clearly. They experience people as *extensions of themselves* rather than as separate individuals with differing needs, desires, and feelings. As such, they assume that their romantic partner wants what they want. Second, they overestimate their own emotional empathy, thereby punishing their supply for not living up to this false narrative. The narcissist demonstrates this through being over the top and dramatic, turning on crocodile tears when they feel the situation calls for it, but if you do not meet them where they are by giving a similar performance, you will be accused of not caring. Third, their defensiveness distorts their perceptions of and interactions with others. They use denial of malicious behaviors, self-entitlement, blame, contempt, criticism, and aggression to ward off shame.

All these issues impair narcissists' capacity to accurately take in another person's reality, including that person's love for them. In fact, narcissists' lack of emotional intelligence allows them to manipulate and exploit others to get what they want while their impaired emotional empathy desensitizes them to the pain they inflict.

This is not to say that they have no attachments to the people that serve them, or that they don't know what empathy looks like, but they do not experience love, morality, empathy, understanding, loyalty, humility, honesty, kindness, integrity, selflessness, or compassion the way healthy people experience these values—especially when it comes to love.

Considering how narcissists love-bomb you, the juxtaposition between what they convey to you and the reality of the matter is dizzying. They portray their love to you as infinite and dreamy when, in fact, it is the opposite. The idea of love is something they exploit and use to get what they want from you.

Love is difficult to measure, but love is defined by psychologist and biologist Enrique Burunata as a physiological motivation, such as hunger, thirst, sleep, and sex drive.[5] One study revealed that participants felt loved by a partner who showed interest in their affairs; gave them emotional and moral support; disclosed intimate facts to them, expressed feelings for them, such as "I'm happier when I'm near you"; and/or tolerated their demands and flaws so as to maintain the relationship. The narcissist can portray themselves in these ways with no feeling whatsoever for the person that they are exploiting. Because cognitive empathy allows them to know what love may look and feel like, the narcissist is able to mimic "passion" in the early stages of the love-bombing phase, and we may mistake this for real connection.

Let's be clear: *This is not true love.* Narcissists may peddle the idea that you are in a loving, empathetic relationship with reciprocity and all good things, but this is always an exploitation of your own projections, your own expectations, and your own ideals of what a relationship could be. As a matter of fact, narcissists mirror your behaviors and tastes so much that you inevitably fall in love with a fake version of your perfect partner, which has been built to suit your own specific desires. **In some ways, the narcissist allows you to fall in love with the *best* version of *yourself* while you, ironically, become the *worst* version of *yourself*.**

That's right! *You*, as the survivor of narcissistic abuse, are the magic and the inspiration in the narcissistic relationship! The narcissist is merely gleaning information from you and creating a wonderful partner based on your expressions of what your ideal partner would be like. They may seem to "become" that person, but this act is unsustainable. In the end, you will have been exploited to provide positive attention and sexual satisfaction that fuels a narcissist's ego and sense of self.

Real love is not only physical romance, and it's not **codependency**. For Aristotle and Saint Thomas Aquinas, it's "to will the good of another."[6] In a healthy union of two individuals, it requires that we see the other person as separate from ourselves. Further, in *The Art of Loving*, Erich Fromm emphasizes that love entails an effort to develop knowledge, responsibility, and commitment.[7] Love involves offering attention, respect, support, compassion, and acceptance, but narcissists aren't motivated to really know and understand others. In fact, oftentimes they are jealous of and in competition with most people around them.

THE JEALOUS NARCISSIST

After reviewing the list of personality traits the narcissist possesses, we might understand that narcissists have little to no moral compass and little to no interest in understanding the damage their actions cause. While they have little regard for others' feelings, they themselves frequently feel negative emotions, such as jealousy.

A 2016 study by Kristi Chin investigated the triggers behind jealousy in narcissists. Chin and her colleagues were specifically looking into romantic narcissistic relationships and found two key reasons behind jealousy within them: entitlement and self-esteem. In fact, there was a correlation between these two points: the lower the narcissist's self-esteem, the higher the probability was that they would be jealous or feel entitled to things, such as money, fame, sex, and attention.[8]

Envy of other people's successes can trigger a narcissistic injury; an example of this scenario might be the narcissistic husband whose wife succeeds in achieving a promotion, or the narcissistic manager whose team member receives personal recognition and praise from the CEO. It's not just the event itself that can trigger envy in the narcissist, but the mere fact that attention is not on them. This is compounded by their lack of empathy, because they have a difficult time feeling or sharing in the joy that others, especially their victims, experience, due to their having put so much energy into devaluing this specific person. Some common signs that a narcissist is envious of you include praising your success initially but then trying to move the focus elsewhere; trying to outdo you; downplaying your successes; or even indicating that it was just luck that got you any achievements. In some instances, they may sabotage your efforts directly or try to take credit for your successes.

When a narcissist becomes covetous or jealous, or feels wounded by another person's success or lack of attention, it is called a *narcissistic injury*, and it's likely to leave the narcissist in a state of low self-esteem. A 2017 study indicated that narcissists try to make others jealous to exact revenge, test their relationship, or gain security within it.[9]

JEALOUSY AND NARCISSISTIC PUNISHMENT

Narcissists may become jealous of others in their lives, or they may lose interest in their narcissistic supply as their expectation of intimacy and devotion increases, or when they've won at their game. As such, many have trouble sustaining a relationship—romantic, platonic, or professional—for more than six months to a few years. They prioritize power over intimacy and loathe vulnerability. As the vulnerability of their supply gets higher, the stakes get higher for the relationship, and the narcissist's mask begins to slip off. That's when the punishment begins.

The narcissist punishes their victims in various ways, and most, if not all, of them are serious. Many of my clients report that they became suicidal after extricating themselves from the narcissist's cult, and that is because their abusers studied them daily and understood their darkest fears.

A jealous narcissist will become your own personal terrorist. If you have children with them, they may harm your children. If you have animals, they may harm your animals. Chillingly, this is often because they can be jealous of children or pets—basically, anything that takes your attention away from them. They will exploit the judicial system and will fracture your professional relationships in ways that could never be repaired.

Most of my clients report that passive aggression and the **silent treatment** were omnipresent forms of punishment for anything their narcissists deemed an injury. The narcissist may practice financial abuse by withholding money from you or may drag you through the legal system using what is called "legal abuse." There is even a term for the aftereffects of legal abuse, "Legal Abuse Syndrome," which is recognized as a form of post-traumatic stress disorder.

Many even use "spiritual abuse," which happens when someone uses spiritual or religious beliefs to hurt, scare, or control you. It can involve someone forcing you or your children to participate in spiritual or religious practices when you don't want to.

They may also practice "reactive abuse," which is when the narcissist will press you so far that you react in front of others, or they record your reaction to be used against you in their smear campaign.

SEXUAL ABUSE

For the narcissist, sexual abuse is used to control your behavior, elevate their feelings of superiority, reenact their fantasies (not yours), and paralyze you. Sexual abuse is one of the most emotionally and psychologically intense weapons at a narcissist's disposal. They begin the abuse by grooming you—performing a mildly abusive act to see whether you acquiesce. For instance, they might fondle you in front of your mother or demand sexting while you are at work. These unwanted or embarrassing sexual acts are designed to catch you off guard and create a feeling of trepidation. They may test the waters with mild strangulation, pinching, slapping, or other degrading practices. It may leave you feeling like a possession or feeling humiliated. If you try to confront them with your perspective, they will minimize, deny, or blame you by bringing up some past issue that you may have shared with them regarding sex.

The narcissist's sexual behaviors are not just taboo, but abusive and extremely dangerous. They may push you to do things that you may have never done, some degrading sexual behavior that you may not have any interest in doing, and they may become violent if you do not obey. They may record you doing this unwanted act, to use the video as leverage against you later on.

The narcissist may give you a sexually transmitted disease (STD) and then tell you that you are now tied to each other through it. They may even give you a disease and then gaslight you into believing that you gave it to them.

Some narcissists will withhold sex as a form of punishment, whereas others will consider a number of times they can exploit their victims, sexually, as a sign of victory. They may even brag about their conquests by using these "stats." Some of my clients have described having sex up to twelve times a day, to keep the narcissist from punishing them. To add insult to injury, they had to listen to their abuser brag about this, indicating the act was not only used as narcissistic punishment against their victim but as one-upmanship against an unknown "rival."

When you first and unknowingly consider a romantic relationship with a narcissist, they may even pretend that they are not interested in moving quickly into a sexual relationship. When you decide to do so, they may tell you that you are an amazing sexual partner, "the best they have ever had," but as soon as you do not deliver what they request of you, they may accuse you of being manipulative, controlling, damaged, or a prude. You will then be criticized for your sexual desires or lack thereof. You may be called a whore or worse over time. They may ask you about past partners and then use that information against you. They may also insist that you participate in threesomes and may accuse you of overdressing or underdressing, flirting, flaunting your body, and cheating, and you will be punished accordingly.

The narcissist may use harassment, guilt, shame, blame, or rage to persuade you into having sex with them. They may insist on sex after an argument, to prove your commitment. This is sexual abuse. They may threaten infidelity if you do not go along with their desires, telling you that they will be "pushed into" cheating. When you think you have pleased them, they turn up that dial again and require more.

Many of my clients describe being with a narcissist as being raped, and this is because they later realize they were being coerced the entire time and therefore unable to give real consent.

NARCISSISM ON A SOCIAL SCALE: FROM CULT LEADERS TO CEOS

When we talk about rape and all the other horrifying practices that antisocial personalities and narcissists partake in, we see this undercurrent of a lack of empathy. We see that individual narcissists are using and abusing their victims, and we see this with cult leaders as well. If a person like this should come into a position of power, a lack of empathy quickly becomes dangerous on a grand scale. From Jonestown to Heaven's Gate, narcissistic cult leaders, which we will discuss in greater depth in Chapter 5, have shown us that a lack of empathy, writ large, can lead to genocide and other monstrosities.

In the NXIVM cult, many young women were exploited, victimized, and branded by their very unassuming cult leader, Keith Raniere. Raniere fancied himself a visionary but, thankfully, a jury in Manhattan disagreed and sentenced him in 2021 to 120 years in prison for racketeering, sex trafficking, and other charges. In this cult, a harem of sexual "slaves" were branded with his initials on their pelvis and coerced into having sex with him. These women were taught to revere him and were ordered to maintain a near-starvation diet to achieve the physique he found desirable. One of the victims was fifteen years old when the abuse began. It took many of the victims years to process what had happened to them and to unravel the web of lies that was fed to them.

The narcissistic cult leader does not always use sexual abuse to punish their victims, as Raniere often did, but time and again, narcissistic jealousy and its continual need for more and more attention lead to serious consequences for the cult leader's victims. Jim Jones's Peoples Temple began innocently enough, helping the poor in Indiana, but by the end, his cult victims ultimately were murdered—whether by cyanide or bullet—the ultimate form of narcissistic punishment.

Not only cult leaders, but narcissists in everyday positions of power and influence can be dangerous as well. Because they have no empathy, the destruction that comes from a narcissist's antisocial actions is pervasive. So many pathological personalities are in C-suites, boardrooms, and war rooms across the globe. Per Jonathan Ronson's book *The Psychopath Test*, 4 percent of CEOs are clinical psychopaths, four times the incidence rate of psychopathy in society at large.[10]

On a macro scale, a narcissist in power can cause severe damage. To me, this drives home how important it is to address how we, as a society, distinguish between healthy personalities and forms of success, and those that might enjoy creating chaos not only in our relationships but in our world.

THERAPY TIP:
DIALECTICAL BEHAVIORAL THERAPY—
WAYS TO HEAL AFTER TRAUMA

- **Meditation.** Meditation can improve mental health, boost your satisfaction at work, enhance your relationships, encourage creativity, decrease anxiety, and help with depression.
- **Aromatherapy and essential oils.** In dialectical behavioral therapy (DBT), we use the five senses to get grounded, and smell is one of my favorites to use for this purpose. Beyond helping ground us during or after triggers, a 2011 study demonstrated that certain fragrances, such as peppermint oil, lower stress and improve overall outlook.[11]
- **Performing acts of kindness.** A simple, daily practice of altruism can dramatically alter your outlook on the world. Particularly, if you are feeling anger, it is good to practice love, such as smiling at a stranger or sending a loving text to a cherished friend. In DBT, we call this "opposite action." You can practice opposite action in different ways. If you are feeling depressed, you should get active. Small things can shift your mood.

Chapter 4

What the Narcissist Will NOT Do

There are days when therapy is exhausting. It can become such heavy work to hold space for people who are spinning and ruminating for many years, dealing with an inability to process so much of what they have endured, but the hardest thing to witness in my amazing clients is the countless communications they have with their narcissistic partner, desperately trying to get their abuser to see things the way they should. The energy that they put out, in efforts to change their partner, is immeasurable. Countless hours of wasted time for decades. I think of my client Ellen, who continues to try to change her abuser. She is exhaustedly communicating ways that she believes he should do this or that—with no effort by him to comply.

A big part of what I provide psychoeducation around is this: It's not that the narcissist "cannot" do things differently. It's that they "will not" do things differently.

———❦———

So far in this book, we've talked about what narcissists do, as well as actions and symptoms that define clinical narcissism. Now, let's talk about what narcissists *won't* do. There are a lot of things they will not do because they think they are above doing them, among a variety of other selfish reasons. This is important ground to cover because it will disabuse you of any harmful misconceptions you might have that a narcissistic abuser will change.

THEY WILL NOT BE HONEST OR AUTHENTIC, EXCEPT FOR THE OCCASIONAL KERNEL OF TRUTH (even a broken clock is right twice a day).

When it comes to coercive control, narcissists understand that they must pepper truths throughout their fraudulent gestures and stories, so as to confuse you. For instance, they may say they have a degree from an illustrious university, and because they seem to be well spoken and have a fake degree hanging on their wall, you believe them. After all, why would anyone feel the need to lie about something like that? Many will also fake a history in law enforcement.

Your rational mind might take such things to be the truth because of the narcissist's carefully laid context clues, but if God himself gives you a résumé, check the references. There is no point in applying logic when it comes to the narcissist. Yes, narcissists are delusional and live in a fantasy world, but it is not often that simple to decipher. This is because narcissists engage in truth distortion frequently, whether by exaggerating the truth and downplaying their lies, or by twisting the truth to serve their agenda. Truth distortion is lying, plain and simple. There are no such things as "my truths." There is the truth or a nontruth. By lying pervasively and for prolonged periods of time, narcissists raise falsehood to an art form that can also be called *proselytizing*, whereby they recruit you to believe their lies so that they can ultimately brainwash and control you.

Narcissists often use **dissociation**—erasing memories or disconnecting from reality—because their contact with the world and with others comes through the fictitious construct of *the false self*. In other words, narcissists never experience reality directly but rather, through a distorted lens. They get rid of any information that challenges their grandiose self-perception or the narrative they have constructed to excuse, and legitimize, their exploitative behaviors, as well as low self-worth.

In an attempt to compensate for the yawning gaps in their memory, narcissists employ **confabulation**—that is, they invent ostensibly plausible scenarios of how things might, could, or should have occurred. To outsiders, these fictional stopgaps may appear to be lies, but to the narcissist, this is what they believe, and that makes it so. These shaky, concocted fillers are subject to frequent revision as the narcissist's inner world and external circumstances evolve. They will create and re-create their "truths" as needed. They are not invested in the emotions and cognitive processes that are integral parts of forming real memories, and the eternally shifting sands of their "truths" can confuse their victims. In fact, they may even apologize when they're caught in a lie, but this is never an apology in earnest, only an apology to confuse.

THEY WILL NOT BE CONSISTENT.

The narcissist's practice of blowing hot and cold goes beyond truth and lies. They seem to change their opinions, plans, and wishes on a daily basis. Their actions almost never match their words. Their impulsivity, coupled with their desire to create chaos and confusion, makes inconsistency their modus operandi (MO). It becomes impossible to find the rationale behind their behavior, much less to figure them out. You might drive yourself insane trying to make sense out of the narcissist's actions, but it is a waste of energy and effort.

The most painful aspect of the narcissist's inconsistency and lack of integrity is that they often make grand promises in their love-bombing and future-faking phases, proposing plans for the future that they know they won't stick to. We tend to believe in their promises, only to ultimately realize that they never intended to act on them. As a result, as survivors of narcissistic abuse, we find ourselves in a regular state of disappointment. I remember this feeling washing over me, like a physical rush of shame; that I was holding space for someone who would only leave me stranded, with a shattered sense of self and a long road to recovery ahead.

THEY WILL NOT BE FAITHFUL, TRUSTWORTHY, OR LOYAL.

Many victims and survivors of narcissistic abuse struggle with this one because the narcissist is so seemingly involved in their life that people often wonder when they would find the time to seek other company, but believe me—*they find the time!*

Narcissists are addicted to attention and treat it the same way they might treat a drug addiction. In other words, they will stop at nothing to get it. They have to have a gaggle of supplemental supplies waiting in the wings, in case they have a moment of disconnect from their main supply.

Additionally, poor impulse control; a big ego; exaggerated feelings of self-importance; delusions of grandeur; and a lack of remorse, empathy, and shame are key reasons that narcissists lie and cheat on their partners. Most of all, they simply think they can get away with it, and they are not wrong. They have a master plan but know that their skills at manipulating and lying will get them through the barriers that may present themselves along the way, and they know this because it generally has worked!

Their means of baiting their next victims are many, but ones my clients and I have run into include dating apps, tantric meetup groups, and making bogus business promises to professionals that they may find themselves around. Narcissists may also frequent brothels and "massage parlors" for supplemental supply. A cheating narcissist is likely to exhibit the following behaviors:

- Disappearing frequently and being vague about their whereabouts.

- Flirting with someone other than their partner. This is a big tell, but because the nature of narcissistic abuse is so insidious, it may be discreet like placing their hand a little to low on someone's back.
- Not putting their phone down or letting you anywhere near it. Almost every narcissist has a burner phone anyway, or more than one alias. Many of them have different names than the one they've shared with you. Many people report to me that they have done background checks on their abuser and learned of the various names that the narcissist went by.
- Accusing you of having an affair. Every accusation from the narcissist is a confession, and they will absolutely tell on themselves when it comes to cheating in this way.
- Experiencing sudden changes in their libido.

If you struggle with this last one, I would err on the side of caution and get a screening for sexually transmitted diseases (STDs). Many clients come to me and share that they were blindsided by the fact that their abuser was cheating on them. Narcissists are gluttons who think they are entitled to sex, or at least attention, all the time. Protect yourself and pay attention to any changes in your anatomy that warrant a doctor's appointment because STDs are common when dealing with a narcissist. Even if you aren't experiencing any physical symptoms, if you can't shake the feeling that your abuser has cheated on you, you owe it to yourself to get tested. Many live with dis-"ease" from this relationship.

THEY WILL NOT BE SATIATED.

No matter what they do, nothing can make them happy—not sex, money, food, success, fame, attention, and/or drugs. Narcissists forever make the mistake of thinking that to win is to feel satiated; they get a rush of pleasure when they "win," but this moment of pleasure is superficial and fleeting. The pleasure the narcissist feels is similar to that of a drug high, and when you get caught up with a narcissist, you will become involved in the highs and lows they experience. If you grew up in a household of ups and downs, you may not recognize the toxicity in this. For them, it's an intensely thrilling but ultimately meaningless experience that leaves them immediately craving the next rush, which is exactly how you will feel after spending any significant amount of time on their roller-coaster ride.

One of the narcissist's fatal flaws is that they can't differentiate between pleasure and happiness. They continue to chase after the former at the expense of the latter, which leaves them emptier and more miserable as time moves on. Remember, the more you try to satiate a narcissist, the more they will turn up the dial of punishment you will receive. The narcissist will always choose dominance over happiness, but happiness comes from feeling settled and soothed and as close to our baseline as possible. The more ups and downs and dysregulation that the narcissist experiences, and the further they get from their baseline, the more traumatic it becomes for them and for everyone around them.

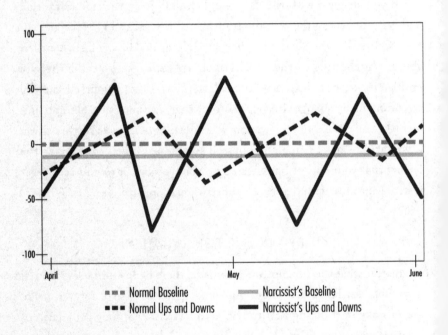

Think about the happiest times in your life. Maybe you were experiencing a connection to nature or to other beings that had you laughing and feeling joyful, or maybe you found yourself helping others or being inspired by others. Happiness comes from being kind and loving; from doing good deeds and being a good person; from feeling a deep sense of connection with others; from making a positive contribution; and from living a meaningful life.

These fractured souls do not feel these emotions the same way we do; narcissists tend to have an agenda, which leads them to an inability to experience emotions in a healthy way. As we discussed when we covered cognitive and affective empathy, there is a difference in their brain that inhibits their emotional intelligence. Imagine living a life without happiness, how angry someone living that life might become to see others who can experience this kind of joy. They would probably blame others for their never being satiated, right? Now, imagine how vengeful that someone may become to others and society as a whole because they can never have what others have. Because they can never "win."

As time goes on, the narcissist becomes increasingly furious and increasingly destructive. This inability to ever feel satiated leads to that ever-expanding inner abyss. I'd feel pity for narcissists in this regard, were it not for the fact that they do so much harm to others.

THEY WILL NOT HELP OTHERS WITHOUT AN AGENDA.

Acting selflessly implies you can identify and work to meet another person's needs without any thought of your own gain. A narcissist does good deeds to get adulation or fame, to make connections or network, to market themselves, to get a tax write-off, to punish others, or to have a sense of superiority and power over others. Giving or helping anonymously removes the reward factor for someone living with NPD, and they may consider it pointless. It's not truly about helping others.

Additionally, by appearing to be giving and helpful, narcissists manage their self-esteem and can make themselves feel superior to others. A narcissist will remind you forever about how much they helped you when you were in need, thereby inducing feelings of guilt in their victim, even accusing you of stealing or peddling a false narrative to others. A narcissistic parent, for example, will use this dynamic with their children, even about things that are normal and expected for a parent to provide, such as clothing, food, and shelter.

Narcissists will also seek positions of power over people in need. That's why you can even find some of them in such fields as teaching, self-help, religion, politics, law, mental health, medical care, and so on. They prey on people who are in need, and they love the power dynamic.

THEY WILL NOT HAVE *TRANSFORMING* INSIGHT INTO WHO THEY ARE.

In a study published in the *Journal of Personality and Social Psychology* in 2012 called "You Probably Think This Paper's About You: Narcissists' Perceptions of Their Personality and Reputation," scientists Carlson, Vazire, and Oltmanns found that people with both subclinical and clinical narcissism understand that they have narcissistic traits and a narcissistic reputation.[1] In other words, even those that are not very symptomatic and therefore cannot be officially diagnosed with NPD know what they are.

They also understand that others do not see them as positively as they see themselves. From the perspective of a narcissist, others fail to perceive the full magnitude of their likability, intelligence, and attractiveness. The discrepancy between their self-perceptions and their meta-perceptions, or fake selves, might explain why narcissists behave in arrogant ways: they may be seeking the recognition they believe they deserve but do not get.

The problem here is that cognitive understanding of one's disorder does not constitute a *transforming* insight. In other words, it has no emotional parallel, and so the narcissist does not internalize what they understand and learn about their disorder. This knowledge does not become a motivating part of the narcissist's life but remains an inert and indifferent piece of knowledge, with minor influence on the narcissist's subconscious.

The narcissist may grow aware of certain behaviors of theirs that are pathological, dysfunctional, or self-defeating and even label them as such, but they never grasp the psychodynamic significance of their conduct, their deeper layers of motivation, and the relentless and unchangeable engine at the serpentine core of their being. They may make admissions about their bad behavior and even apologize, but they will not study its origin and are unlikely to work toward making changes.

Narcissists seldom change, and they definitely rarely heal. In other words, they can practice new behaviors, but they will not change their behaviors. It is a rigid disorder. The neuroplasticity in their brain—the ability of their brain to create new pathways—seems to be limited. Generally, when a narcissist finds themselves in therapy, their emphasis is more on pointing the finger at the people that have been harmed by them and less about they, themselves, changing. It is, in part, because most do not want to change. I believe it would take inpatient treatment for a prolonged period of time for a narcissist to change. Some clients come to me after thirty years in a relationship with a narcissist who promised, the entire time, to change.

THEY WILL NOT BE COOPERATIVE.

Narcissists are not prone to being forgiving, ungrudging, unthreatening, or looking to resolve conflict. Because the narcissist overestimates their emotional intelligence, they do not usually see any need to cooperate. Being cooperative would mean an open willingness to learn and collaborate with others, which the narcissist is not interested in doing. They believe that they are the mentor/teacher and everyone should learn from *them*! We see their inability to cooperate mostly in the courtroom if they are asked to co-parent. Co-parenting brings about some unique challenges that take cooperative thinking to overcome. Things like splitting time for custody or the holidays can be difficult for even the most agreeable parents, but narcissists are not among them. Not only are they terrible at this; they also make it hellish to agree on the smallest of issues. They enjoy the chaos they cause in developing co-parenting schedules. They will often-times not agree to custody or other arrangements, much less act nice or agreeable for your child's sake, and will often interfere with your child's routine, appointments, and belongings. It's their way or the highway.

THEY WILL NOT HAVE FOLLOW-THROUGH.

The narcissist is "clickbait," personified. They throw a bunch of things out there to prospects and then seldom deliver on anything. Once a narcissist is found out, they move on, leaving a trail of broken promises in their wake.

A narcissist wants new conquests to believe that they, the abuser, had been the "victim" or the "wounded party" in any previous breakups. They will lavishly embellish their own good qualities as they enthusiastically vilify their exes. They approach this initial stage of the relationship as though they're in a movie.

The narcissist's inability to follow through is partly because, when you are out of sight from a narcissist, you are out of mind. This could be as simple as their promising to call you later in the day and then failing to make the phone call, or it could be as extreme as discussing having a marriage and kids together, without any intention of having a lasting relationship.

Over time, as the victimized partner loses their perfect image in the narcissist's mind, the narcissist will begin to "devalue" the partner, which can involve putdowns, withdrawal of affection, or a discard. Instead of following through on promises, the narcissist disengages, abuses, and may find a new supply.

THEY WILL NOT EMBRACE YOUR AUTONOMY.

The narcissist would rather throw up or break out in hives than congratulate someone on a success. If they do it, look out—they will surely punish that person later. They are pathologically envious and will find ways to detract from your successes or use them against you in some way.

They will minimize your autonomy and independence, deflate it, or ignore it altogether. They may say things like "I need you," so as to make you feel codependent on them. Once they have you locked into codependency, they will take up so much of your energy that you will no longer have time to do things that are important to you. Instead, you will become an extension of them.

A healthy person will celebrate your independent dreams and goals, whereas a narcissist becomes highly threatened by them and will work to undermine you as if their legal name is "Captain Sabotage." When they aren't the center of attention, a narcissist will practice a constant redirection to themselves until they are. This might mean the narcissist readily takes credit for your successes. They may tell others that they paid for your schooling when you put yourself through college; they might let you know that it is because of them that you are feeling anything good. You may notice that your partner simply doesn't bring up to others some tremendous accomplishment that you have just completed.

THEY WILL NOT SUPPORT YOUR INCLUSION OF FRIENDS AND FAMILY.

One of the first things a narcissist does is isolate their supply from family and friends. They want you to be completely dependent on them and eliminate any outside support system you have in place. The more isolated they can get you from friends and family, the easier it is to fool you into believing their narrative, because your friends and family members are the biggest threat to your seeing who the narcissist really is.

It often starts slowly, with their making comments that they do not like your friends or family. The narcissist is well versed in innuendo, inference, passive aggression, and sarcasm. They may drop hints in a way that may even slip under your radar, such as an eye roll.

From there, the abuser's tactics will ramp up. Some of the ways they achieve the goal of isolation include a "divide and conquer" or triangulating approach, such as setting up members of the family against one another or favoring one child over the other. They will also create a competitive and threatening atmosphere and use their flying monkeys or other enablers to back them up. These scenarios often have members of the family or cult vying for the narcissist's approval, or at the very least, trying to keep themselves safe from an attack by the narcissist.

Narcissists are the ultimate puppeteers and will corrupt any environment so that it best serves themselves, with no regard for the pain they cause along the way.

THEY WILL NOT BE SECURE.

Most of us have our own insecurities, but the narcissist lives in a world built entirely around trying to fill that void. Healthy people are not as driven by competition because it is not necessary for them to compete with others. Meanwhile, narcissists are not only competitive but vindictive. They enjoy bringing others down, whereas the secure person *avoids* bringing others down and is more uplifting.

Insecure narcissists may spend a lifetime trying to get vindication for the smallest error. If a narcissist burns a meal, they blame the stove. Secure people will ride out any storm and deal with issues as they arise, but the insecure person will run from things that scare them.

Similarly, securely attached humans approach relationships cooperatively. They work together to achieve shared goals, seek and give each other validation, share accurate and truthful information, and express affection and vulnerability to build trust. There may be conflict, but mutual support is the foundation of the relationship, and respect and love are not at stake whenever there's an argument. In extreme contrast, the person with NPD has an antagonistic and **disorganized attachment style**, which is a relationship in which someone benefits at the expense of another (for more on attachment styles, see pages 184–188).

Common forms of antagonism in the animal kingdom are predation and parasitism. *Predation* is when a predator typically kills and eats its prey to gain life-giving energy. A predatory human relationship may end in murder, but more often, there is a condition of ongoing domination and subjugation because narcissists view all relationships as a struggle for dominance. It's a game of "cat and mouse." They emotionally and perhaps also physically and sexually oppress, intimidate, and violate others to experience and maintain feelings of power and control. Narcissistic displays of dominance may include flagrant forms of aggression, such as hitting, pushing, berating, name-calling, and criticism, or may be more passive-aggressive maneuvers, such as dismissal, the silent treatment, backhanded compliments, jokes at your expense, veiled threats, **breadcrumbing** (leading someone on with mixed messages), and triangulation. Whatever the strategy and however well it is rationalized or disguised, the purpose is to bully the other person into submission.

Between humans, *parasitism* shows up as an exploitative relationship, usually with the parasitic narcissist manipulating or coercing the other person (the host) into providing ongoing resources, such as money, housing, privilege, social standing, sex, and caretaking, among other forms of service. To make this happen more easily, the narcissist uses such tactics as isolation, shame, seduction, fawning, and gaslighting while employing forms of **intermittent reinforcement**, which are very Pavlovian, to create the illusion of reciprocity in the relationship. The relationship not only drains the host of physical and emotional resources but it also alienates that host of their own self-preserving instincts and ability to maintain boundaries.

THEY WILL NOT PUT OTHER PEOPLE FIRST.

Narcissistic entitlement refers to a belief that one's importance, superiority, or uniqueness should result in getting special treatment and receiving more resources than others. It is because of this that a narcissist will not put others before themselves, including their own children. For example, individuals high in narcissistic entitlement think that they should get more respect, more money, and more credit for doing the same work as everyone else. Narcissistic entitlement also includes a willingness to demand this special treatment or extra resources. In a relationship, the narcissist is king or queen.

THEY WILL NOT STOP DEFLECTING
AND PROJECTING.

Finally, when faced with indisputable proof of their wrongdoing, such as receipts, photos, and emails, a narcissist will want to redirect attention back onto you as a distraction. Deflection can include *indirect or nonanswers* (e.g., circular conversations); bringing unrelated details or old issues (particularly your prior "offenses") into the mix; *guilt-tripping* ("After everything I've done for you, this is how you repay me?"); and the all-time favorite of the narcissist—*projection*, accusing you of exactly what they are doing.

When it comes to what a narcissist will and will not do, keep in mind that they will change their behaviors depending upon what they think you may or may not need from them, so as to fulfill what they see as your purpose: providing them with a steady supply of attention. There is always an agenda with a narcissist, and while that agenda may not make sense to rational, healthy minds, it always boils down to fulfilling the narcissist's own insatiable needs and punishing you for getting in their way.

DBT EXERCISE: RADICAL ACCEPTANCE

So many of us have experienced feelings of guilt or shame for having tolerated narcissistic abuse, but I would like to offer you a new tool for your toolbox. We can practice radical acceptance around what we have endured.

Radical acceptance is a therapy practice—a part of dialectical behavioral therapy (DBT)—based on the notion that suffering comes not directly from pain, but from one's attachment to the pain.

Radical acceptance suggests that nonattachment is the key to overcoming suffering. **Nonattachment does not mean not feeling emotions, nor does it mean that you're approving of what happened to you.** Instead, it refers to an intention to not allow your present pain to turn into further suffering. This can help us break free of emotions related to that kind of suffering, such as anger, sadness, and bitterness. Many of my clients find this exercise liberating—even my own therapist has me regularly practice radical acceptance.

If you feel ready to try out radical acceptance, hold your hands in front of you, palms up, and say, "It is what it is." Lift your shoulders in a shrug. Give a half smile and think about accepting what has happened as something you do not have control over and that you cannot spend any more energy trying to change. You didn't *cause* it. You can't *control* it and you cannot *cure* it.

Being a victim is not your fault. It is not your fault that you met a monster. You can now accept that which you cannot control because agonizing over such things and trying to change them adds no value to your life. Remember that all the good things that you thought you fell in love with were actually all the things *you* possess that the narcissist was reflecting back to you—your thoughtfulness, humor, charm, and authenticity. You are the magic and always were. It's time to reclaim it.

Chapter 5

A Cult of One

The phone rings on a Thursday night. John explains through his gasping for air and crying that he has just left what he thinks was a cult. "What is happening to me?" he begs. When I first started doing this work, I would almost think people were prank calling me because it was so hard to believe. When we meet in my office the next day, he tells me that he was love-bombed into a cult and then manipulated for nine years into recruiting others to become involved with an abusive cult leader who would devalue him regularly. So many of us think that cults happen "over there" or to someone far away; no one we know could ever fall victim. Yet so many of my clients have been lured into a devastating cult of one.

⸺⚬⚬⚬⸺

I often talk about narcissistic relationships as "a cult of one." The main purpose of this book is to highlight the sameness between being in a small cult of one, of a few, or of many, because cults are synonymous with domestic abuse and there are important corollaries; so even if you think, "*cults aren't relevant to me,*" I encourage you to read this chapter for some bigger context. In this chapter, we will discuss the cycle of narcissistic abuse within the confines of the cult of many—from luring and recruitment, through **capture-bonding** and manipulation, to indoctrination and brainwashing. There are no *real* differences between a cult of one in an intimate partner relationship with an abuser and a cult of many in a larger group. This chapter is designed to shine a light on the likenesses between the pathology of a cult leader and a narcissist.

When we talk about narcissists in the context of cults, we are not only talking about one-on-one interpersonal relationships but also about religious cults, commercial cults (e.g., pyramid and multilevel marketing schemes), political cults (e.g., the Nazi Party, terrorist organizations), and other groups using coercive control. There may even be cults you have never considered, such as self-help and counseling cults, in which the gurus keep their clients dependent on them while they extract money from their bank accounts for endless and unnecessary sessions.

The strategies that narcissists instinctively use to get their way in personal relationships can be strikingly similar to the coercive tactics used by destructive cult leaders to indoctrinate and control their followers. According to Robert J. Lifton, there are three primary defining characteristics to a cult leader, and I think you will find these familiar because they are tantamount to the characteristics we see in a narcissist. Cult leaders are defined by:

- A charismatic leader who increasingly becomes an object of worship
- Thought reform or coercive control
- Exploitation of its members[1]

In a relationship with a narcissist or in a cult, outsiders are viewed as dangerous or as potential enemies. This turns your red-flag radar outward, distracting you from problems within the narcissistically abusive relationship or cult until it is too late. Viewing others as "the enemy" or "not evolving" can be used to justify a cult's extreme actions, because of the supposed dangers that outsiders pose. From there, cult leaders inject shame, guilt, coercion, and fear to keep their members (victims) in-line. Victims are taught to discount their own intuition and healthy instincts in favor of the narcissist's value system. Over time, victims can lose touch with their own healthy habits and innate values. Having doubts about the cult of one is considered a betrayal and could be met with punishment because the righteousness of the narcissist cult leader is paramount. Closeness to the cult leader is rewarded, but independence is punished. Temporary ostracism, such as passive aggression or the silent treatment, as well as more aggressively violent tactics, are used to punish behavior that doesn't conform to the "rules." Sound familiar? If you are or were in a relationship with a narcissist, I'm betting it does.

Both in a cult and in an individual relationship with a narcissist, lies are repeated so often that they seem true. I've seen people who are unable to discern fact from fiction when they leave cults or these relationships because they were gaslit and brainwashed into believing things that were disconnected from reality. Oftentimes, cult leaders will use repetition or get their members to make false statements so frequently that their victims begin to question accuracy. They often do this through song and music, on repeat, to cement it into the wiring of their victims' brain.

Cult leaders spend their energy creating a scenario where their victims cannot find the truth and end up looking to them for the answers. The problem is, the answers they provide are agenda-driven lies.

CULT ABUSE IS DOMESTIC VIOLENCE

Cult abuse is also a form of domestic violence and coercive control. When you hear the saying "Well, they certainly drank the Kool-Aid," you may think that someone is willingly following another person's lead, but this turn of phrase really blames the person that is being coerced.

The expression actually refers to the Reverend Jim Jones, who killed 918 people in Jonestown in 1978 when he coerced them into drinking cyanide-laced Kool-Aid. "Drank the Kool-Aid" suggests these people died by suicide when, in fact, they were murdered by Jones. A lot of my clients express to me a concern that they were being poisoned by their abuser or the minions of their abuser, with the abuser sometimes accusing *them* of doing the poisoning, but the irony is that the narcissist is "poison personified."

What does this have to do with domestic abuse? Well, if you think about it, cult leaders and narcissists both prove themselves to be domestic abusers, through such shared practices as:

- Keeping people unaware of what is going on outside of the cult
- Controlling their environments at all times
- Systematically creating a sense of powerlessness in their victims
- Creating a system of rewards and punishments to diminish a person's former identity
- Manipulating the victim's social environment to solidify the narcissist's ideology
- Creating a closed system of logic and an authoritarian structure that doesn't permit feedback

It simply does not matter what the group supports or what the narrative becomes.

It isn't about religion. It is about control. As a matter of fact, the more peculiar the ideology is, the more the victim must have been manipulated, and therefore, the more the narcissistic cult leader thrives. They may think, *"If I can get them to brand one another with my initials, I really can get them to do anything I choose. I am a god to them."* Keith Raniere, from the NXIVM cult, was able to get his followers to do just that. Many of my clients were coerced into getting tattoos as well, a different kind of branding and a way that the cult leader or narcissist can gauge a victim's devotion.

In an intimate relationship, it is no different. The narcissist is charming, gets you to pull away from your support system, and then begins to intimidate and manipulate you. When that control is lost, some abusers take drastic, even lethal, measures to regain power over their victims.

When you can see that the tactics of the narcissist and the cult leader are the same, and understand that these tactics are used as a means of domestic violence, you can begin to see the trauma that you may have endured and move toward protecting yourself and healing. It is in this understanding that you can become free.

TYPES OF CULT LEADERS

Cult leaders are often narcissists who failed in their quest to "be something" or to become famous. They impose on their victims an exclusionary or inclusionary shared psychosis replete with persecutory delusions, imagined enemies, mythical and/or grandiose narratives, and apocalyptic scenarios.

In an article, Rachel Bernstein, an esteemed colleague and a California-based therapist who works with former cult members, describes a cult leader as feeling as though they are entitled to completely lie to you—to put on this good, charming face—to get you to believe what they're selling, whatever it is, whether it's God or a product or anything. The cult-leading narcissist, she says, is a "bottomless pit of ego need."[2] Let's talk about what some versions of cult leaders may look like.

The types of cult leaders include:

The Above-the-Law Narcissist. As the leader of their congregation (even if it's a congregation of one), this narcissist feels entitled to special amenities and benefits not accorded to the "rank and file." They expect to be waited on by their servants. The narcissist also feels above the law, and this, along with the idea that they have fooled both their followers and law enforcement, leads to criminal acts, incestuous or nonconsensual polygamous relationships, and recurrent friction with the authorities.

In the HBO docuseries *The Vow*, the creators chronicle how NXIVM cult leader Keith Raniere was able to first sell self-improvement courses as a multilevel marketing scheme, then use his courses to brainwash followers into providing blackmail against themselves, branding themselves with his initials, and having sex with him. Raniere was arrested on several charges, including sex trafficking, in June 2019, but before that, he captured hundreds of followers over decades with his charismatic personality and teachings. He accepts no accountability, to this day, as is the case for most narcissists.[3]

The Delusional Narcissist. According to Bernstein, who has worked with eight former members from NXIVM, a delusional cult leader is the most dangerous kind because they can use their unyielding beliefs to convince others to buy into the delusion. She uses the example of Heaven's Gate, a cult where thirty-nine members committed mass suicide as instructed by leader Marshall Applewhite in 1997. Applewhite was convinced a UFO would soon come to Earth and help humans leave their body for a higher existence. Bernstein says, "There is the sense that the leader wasn't trying to get money out of them and he wasn't trying to use them. He really believed that this mothership was coming and that they all needed to leave their corporeal existence and go to this mothership, and they all joined in the psychosis."[4] This group-oriented delusion is a diagnosable condition called **shared psychotic disorder**, according to the National Institutes of Health,[5] which we will discuss again later in this chapter. While we may not have a shared psychotic disorder, many of my clients report doing the dirty work of their abusers and following them blindly, even helping them victimize their former supplies.

The Charismatic Narcissist. There are other ways that narcissists exploit people, as in the case of "the preacher-turned-egomaniac." This type of cult leader may start as a teacher, street preacher, or in another public-speaking position. Eventually, they realize people cling onto what they have to say and they decide to run with that skill. This is the self-declared "guru," and they could be a guru of anything. They "suddenly realize that everyone listens to everything they say, and they are pied pipers, and people will do things just because they told them to do it. And they start to morph into this kind of ego maniacal monster," Bernstein says.[6]

Jim Jones was one of these types. Jones started as a religious preacher and eventually had thousands of followers at his organization, the Peoples Temple, in California. Jones convinced more than a thousand followers to move with him to a Guyanese jungle encampment he called "Jonestown."

When a member of the US Congress arrived at Jonestown to investigate the operation, Jones told his followers to drink Kool-Aid that had been laced with cyanide, and more than nine hundred of them did. This was called a mass suicide, but was it?

The ones who refused to drink the cyanide cocktail were shot to death or forcibly injected with the cyanide. This is so important to highlight because many people think of cult followers as lemmings, but many people who have tried to leave cults don't necessarily die by suicide. They may die by homicide, as Jones's members did, at the hands of a cruel narcissist who can't bear to see them go. The homicide may even be gradual as the strictures put in place by the cult-leading narcissist cause the victim's health to fail, which is also what happens when you live with a narcissist. Your health will fail.

— ∞ —

There is a pattern that cult leaders and narcissists follow; Part 2 of this book goes more in depth into the cycle that the cult leader enacts and progressively engages in: recruitment, manipulation, indoctrination, and destruction:

STEP 1. RECRUITMENT

The narcissist's cult is missionary and imperialistic, forever seeking new recruits. They may hook people with the promise of a business opportunity. They may woo a new supply or cult member by pretending to be attentive, compassionate, empathic, flexible, self-effacing, and helpful, and they train their existing followers to be like this too. At home, though, among the "veteran" members, they are tyrannical, demanding, opinionated, aggressive, and exploitative.

Love-bombing in cults is a coordinated effort, usually under the direction of leadership, which involves long-term members' flooding recruits and newer members with flattery and verbal attention to get them to join and go deeper into the cult. A good example of this might be the communal narcissist or cult leader getting their validation, admiration, and reassurance from helping other people—but only when there is an audience to witness their "good-heartedness."

What this means is they often come off as really good people others want to associate themselves with, but this is all a superficial front. They will inspire you to be the best version of yourself and to spread that to others. This could manifest in the form of helping out on the weekends at your local homeless shelter or going all the way to a developing nation to be of assistance there. But as you work your way up the ranks of the cult and provide more collateral, the mask will slip, and you will come under assault from the communal narcissist's game of brainwashing, gaslighting, and other forms of manipulation.

Cult leaders and narcissists alike do not have a particular "type" they look for when they're recruiting new members; instead, they seek victims with little regard for anything besides the recruit's compliance and potential to be groomed. For this reason, narcissists may be attracted to people in vulnerable situations, as well as people pleasers and approval seekers, as new sources of supply.

People pleasers, approval seekers, or codependents are the perfect prey because they have a deep-seated emotional need to feel secure, a feeling they have learned only comes from making sure others are happy and satisfied. These emotional needs may stem from trauma or neglect, but regardless of their source, they manifest as an intense need to please others at the expense of the people pleaser's own happiness. Although being generous and helpful makes us feel happy, people-pleasing behavior, or living in servitude, can be problematic because it leads to compliance or conformity at the expense of setting up healthy boundaries, which makes us more vulnerable to being victimized by narcissists.

Many of my clients do not necessarily feel that they are this way and many are not; even so, the vast majority had not developed healthy boundaries by the time they encountered a narcissist, which left them vulnerable to abuse.

Because our society places very different external expectations on men and women, people pleasing may help explain why many survivors of narcissistic and/or cult abuse are women. Usually described as "gender roles" or "gender norms," some of the behaviors we learn from childhood can make women particularly susceptible to the dangers of people pleasing. Young girls are told to be quiet and pleasant, to be orientated toward others, to not speak up for what they want, and to please others. These gender-based stereotypes are continuously reinforced in our society in a manner that distinctly disadvantages women, and as a result, women are suffering from more victimization.

Beyond gender norms, something to consider is that spiritual abuse on any level is connected to the narcissistically abusive relationship. Apart from cults, many mainstream belief systems expect servitude and blind loyalty from their members, thereby priming them for the possibility of victimization inside or outside the organization. In other words, even if your place of worship is not toxic, its teachings may have contributed to your being victimized by others. This is because being discouraged to think for themselves and being encouraged to implicitly follow strong, charismatic personality types makes people vulnerable to abuse from a narcissist.

STEP 2: MANIPULATION

The narcissist and the cult leader both insist on blind acceptance of and loyalty to their rules and preferences. The narcissistic cult leader may think they are king, but the truth is their followers are being led by a fretful child. They have created an alternate reality, their "own little world," if you will, and that is the reality their "followers" must accept without question. Before their followers can doggedly adhere to their belief system, though, they must often be manipulated into doing so. As with the individual narcissist, this manipulation begins insidiously before ramping up into more overt tactics.

Capture-Bonding and Increased Isolation. After a narcissist has stalked, recruited, or lured their supply, they generally move on to love-bombing, which looks like capture-bonding in the cult cycle of abuse. In capture-bonding, the victim, motivated by the cult's allegedly loving mission, engages in such dangerous practices as giving away their material possessions, changing their clothing or their hairstyle to match the cult's "uniform," moving into the cult's compound, and possibly changing their name. In an abusive relationship, you may have noticed changes in your mannerisms, attire, and overall presentation. Gradually, the narcissistic cult leader will isolate their victims until they are dependent on them emotionally, sexually, financially, and socially.

The narcissistic cult leader closely monitors and censors information from the outside, exposing their captive audience only to select data and analyses. We see this often with narcissists and social media. They may take over their victims' email addresses or Instagram accounts to keep them from receiving any information that they feel would expose the truth about them. In the scenario where the narcissist or cult leader is in the public eye, they may use nondisclosure agreements (NDAs) to keep their victims from sharing their stories of abuse.

Rules, Regulations, and Micromanagement. Once the new recruit is sturdily ensconced within the community, the narcissistic cult leader's mask of love and compassion begins to slip and their true desire for manipulation and control glares through. A common way manipulation and control first demonstrate themselves is through the hyperspecific rules and responsibilities a cult leader assigns to their followers. They will keep you so busy and distracted, it goes unnoticed.

The narcissistic cult leader is as micromanaging as they are charismatic, exerting control over the minutest details and behaviors of their followers and punishing anyone who withholds information or fails to conform to their wishes, goals, and whims. They have boundaries for their own private lives but often deny privacy to their adherents. Even innocuous activities, such as meeting a friend or visiting one's family, require their permission because this is considered a threat to their "control bubble." They may control everything down to a follower's bathing habits.

Some of the cult leader's rules and preferences will be around basic, intimate needs like eating and sleeping; they will use sleep deprivation and caloric reduction/promotion to manipulate their victims, all under the guise of love and care. If a follower presses back on these extreme rules, the cult leader will foment such doubt in their ability to self-manage that they may give in to these gaslighting tactics.

Many who have had the fortunate experience of getting out of a cult or a narcissistically abusive relationship report their abuser waking them when they were sleeping or insisting upon certain dietary practices.

Overt Manipulation and Punishment. Beyond rules and regulations, the sky's the limit for mind games, gaslighting, and confusion. In the case of NXIVM, Keith Raniere blackmailed his victims, a gathering of information that he called collecting "collateral." He would demand explicit photos and information from his followers, and then threaten to expose the information to their family, friends, or the public at large, to keep them obeying his wishes. This was itself a form of manipulation, and the stakes got higher and higher with each piece of collateral he collected from them. He often told them that if they were really serious about their devotion, they would up the ante with what they were willing to share with him. In the cult of one, you may be recorded, sometimes without knowledge, for collateral.

When manipulation and gaslighting don't work, or if you try to challenge the narcissist's narrative in any way, you may be met with serious punishment, such as physical or verbal abuse. Take, for example, what many narcissists do when they interact with subordinates in business. When hiring, they look for applicants who only have lesser educations, because they believe that they will have an easier time molding them into whatever they want them to be.

However, just as survivors of narcissistic abuse state that much of the psychological torment that remains came from covert narcissistic behaviors, punishments that are emotionally or mentally abusive tend to do more damage than physical or verbal abuse. In this case, the abuser causes a great deal of stress and then swoops in to remedy this anxiety in their victim, reinforcing the idea that they are the victim's one true savior.

Manipulation via Use of Other Cult Members. Whereas the individual narcissist's "flying monkeys" are friends and family they have duped into believing them, the narcissistic cult leader's henchmen are built into the fabric of their organization. They are not very dissimilar.

The cult leader might commission others in the group to perpetuate their narratives and make you think that you must be crazy to want to defy them. After all, everyone else is doing what your leader has decided is best for them, and they're fine! Narcissists use this numbers game frequently and will even state that everyone is against you to make you fall in-line.

They might use other cult members as sources of intel on defiant cult members, or they may use the rest of the cult to get to play the victim.

Again, the tactics some narcissists use to get their way in personal relationships can be strikingly similar to the coercive tactics used by destructive cult leaders. They all love-bomb, future-fake, lie, gaslight, project, withhold, triangulate, isolate, intimidate, and manipulate so they can confuse and control you into meeting their needs. The fact that you are outnumbered can make it almost impossible to get away from, because you see the data that so many people are believing them so *you* must be the problem.

STEP 3. INDOCTRINATION

After the cult follower has been isolated, micromanaged, and manipulated, brainwashing and indoctrination are easier for their abuser to perpetrate.

Beyond sharing in their beliefs, indoctrinated followers are easy and profoundly hostile weapons cult leaders can turn on their critics, the authorities, institutions, their personal enemies, or the media if they try to uncover their actions and reveal the truth. During Charles Manson's trial for the Sharon Tate–Leno LaBianca murders, when he arrived in court with a bloody X carved into his forehead, to show he had "X'd himself from your world," the three female Manson Family members also on trial gave themselves similar wounds.

This phenomenon of trauma bonding explains why victims of emotional abuse experience such loyalty to their abuser and we will talk about trauma bonding at length in a later chapter.

STEP 4. DESTRUCTION

Unfortunately, every cult ends in death, whether actual biological death or the figurative (spiritual/psychological) death of the victim.

The Figurative Death of the Cult Abuse Survivor. If you dare try to decamp from a cult, you will be confronted with what we know in the domestic violence space as postseparation abuse, which will be covered in later chapters. You are at your most vulnerable when you finally get away from the cult leader or narcissist. This is the ultimate act of betrayal to them, so they will intimidate, threaten, and abuse the judicial system to further torture you.

Many of my clients share that, after they left, their abuser threatened to "destroy" them. Narcissists will often work toward fulfilling that promise for decades. They and their flying monkeys may try to kill you or harm your career and interpersonal relationships in ways that you could not imagine. This is exactly what a narcissistic cult leader does when a member tries to escape their clutches.

We saw this with actress Leah Remini after she removed herself from the Church of Scientology in 2003. Since then, she has become well known in Hollywood circles as a courageous whistleblower who has publicly condemned the church and remains committed to outing cults as massively abusive organizations. She and cohost Mike Rinder, himself a former high-ranking member of Scientology's Sea Org, created and executive-produced *Leah Remini: Scientology and the Aftermath,* a documentary series. Remini also published a best-selling memoir about her experience, *Troublemaker: Surviving Hollywood and Scientology.*[7] She gives voice to victims in her own story of recovery.

Remini regularly receives threats from lawyers and on social media from the cult she has famously worked to expose. Similarly, Mike Rinder has been labeled a "suppressive person" by the organization and does not have any contact with his two older children or his first wife, who chose to stay behind in the cult of Scientology. After you leave a relationship with a narcissist, you will meet the exact same fate; the attempt to destroy your entire life.

The Threat of Literal Death. Ultimately, the narcissist pays the price for the years of vindictive punishment they've doled out to everyone around them, not to mention their constant demands for attention, adulation, and affirmation. People get tired of the overbearing presence of the narcissist in their lives, of their disruptive influence, and of the damage they do to communities. According to studies of Sun Myung Moon's cult, the Unification Church, the majority of cult members wake from their stupor and are extremely upset due to the high level of fraud they have endured. This upset and departure of the supply negatively impacts the narcissist, of course, and in the setting of a cult, this can mean dire and fatal consequences for the followers that remain.

Earlier, we mentioned the term "shared psychotic disorder," which is when a narcissist or cult leader brainwashes their supply to the point that their supply becomes totally enveloped in the abuser's delusions.

This disorder is what often proves fatal for many narcissistic cults. When one of the partners opts out of their shared psychotic disorder or the mask falls and the truth is fully revealed, the other half feels annulled, incomplete or amputated, and cast out. If this other half is the cult leader, they are likely to react with a depressive episode in which severity and duration can be extreme, as in the cases of so many cult leaders, such as Marshall Applewhite, Jim Jones, David Koresh (head of the Branch Davidians), and others, who saw the organization they'd built crumbling around them and decided they (and their followers) were better off dead than proven wrong.

It is extremely important to understand that narcissists and cult leaders are not easy to spot. On first meeting a narcissist, unless you are already familiar with narcissistic behavior, you are never going to suspect how dangerous they are. They present themselves well; they seem bright and interesting. You will find them to be everyday people just like yourself. They appear to have a lot in common with you: to share your views, values, ideas, and so on. They seem to be very interested in you and have a knack for making you feel as if you are the only person in the room that matters to them.

The reality is they are not like you.

Now that you have a "Narcissism 101" primer and know what to look out for from narcissists, let's move into a discussion of what it's like to live with a narcissist, coping strategies for any time you may still have to spend with them, and key steps to take as you make your escape.

THERAPY TIP: DISTRACTION

Sometimes, when it comes to coping with the stress of dealing with the reality of what this is, distraction can help get our mind out of the spiral of ruminating thoughts that we may be experiencing due to trauma.

If you are feeling particularly overwhelmed, it may help to do something to temporarily distract yourself from the distressing situation until you are able to deal with it calmly. Distraction can involve physically leaving a location, calling a friend or family member, watching a show, reading a book, playing with a pet, or exercising.

Although distraction is not a permanent solution, it can give your nervous system a break and help you return to a calm and level baseline more quickly.

You can also revisit the Radical Acceptance practice (page 62). This content can be difficult to work through; be compassionate to yourself.

Chapter 6

Living with a Narcissist

I remember going out with friends one night, and I was so scared to be out that I even told the others at the table that I was only allowed to sit next to women. My dear friends Yvonne and Duane went along with it, even positioning another friend, Nancy, between Duane and me. We tried to make the best of the evening with several friends, but nobody at the table knew the fear I had about returning home to a person that was sure to punish me for being autonomous and spending time with friends, especially since there were men at the table—which I feared would surely be problematic.

—∞—

There are several different ways victims find themselves cohabitating with a narcissist, but the primary situations include living with a narcissistic partner, parent, or sibling. Many of their characteristics are the same, but before we focus on the narcissistic romantic partner, let's talk a little about the narcissistic parent or sibling.

Narcissistic parents are the groomers who involve their children in sports, pageantry, acting, or cheerleading, and often not because the child wants to participate in them. Other things they may do include:

- Brag about their child to others, but only about superficial things
- Act immature and selfish, oftentimes *parentifying* the child
- Make the child feel bad for not doing what they want done immediately
- Make the child feel guilty by boasting about how much they have done for them, and attribute the child's successes to themselves
- Make the child feel anxious when they know the narcissistic parent is coming home
- Not be around for the child's significant life events or illnesses
- Force the child who does not wish to, to engage in sports or other activities
- Fail to provide warmth and emotional nurturance
- Use them for personal gain
- Become bothered or annoyed when the child needs time and attention
- Get jealous of other family members' interest in the child
- Dangle carrots and future-fake with college payments, help with wedding planning, car payments, or other forms of financial blackmail
- Triangulate siblings against one another or the other parent
- Bad-mouth the child to extended family members
- Go through the child's personal belongings
- Force the child to be their plus-one or to tag along, even if it is for small trips to the store
- Exploit the list of chores and force the child to be their servant
- Belittle the child and their friends when they think their behavior does not fit their superficial narrative
- Refer to themselves in the third person
- Disappear or act out on holidays or birthdays
- Physically punish the child

So many of these characteristics are reported by the partners of narcissists, but the children of narcissists have an incredibly difficult road ahead. This is because they have fewer options to get away from living with their abusive family member, and have a harder time developing their own identity. The narcissist usually has a "**golden child**" who is the favorite; the "**scapegoat child**," the one that gets blamed for everything and internalizes it; and the "**lost child**" who doesn't seem to matter to the narcissist and will try to keep a low profile.

Narcissists with children typically select a golden child who serves as a projection screen for all the positive things they wish to see in themselves. As an above-reproach extension of the narcissist, the golden child is shielded from consequences, praised lavishly by the narcissist, and elevated above other family members. This child is exploited and can exemplify all that the narcissist wanted to be and could not.

The scapegoat is the shadow side of the narcissist, representing the latter's underlying feelings of inadequacy and self-loathing. Scapegoats serve as receptacles for everything the narcissist wishes to disown and throw away about themselves, and they are routinely burdened with excessive responsibility, arbitrary blame, and punishing rage.

Neither the golden nor the scapegoated child is actually seen for who they are or allowed to freely express their authentic, individual selves. They are mere projections in a movie that the narcissist scripts, directs, and stars in. This is the main reason that the children of narcissists suffer from the worst trauma; they are disallowed from ever forming their own identity. In short, they are set up to fail.

The **lost child** is the forgotten child and will sometimes shrink themselves throughout their lives to stay off the radar of their abusive parent, due to the neglect and fear that they feel.

Additionally, when you grow up in a toxic environment, you may internalize it and not develop good coping mechanisms to express your feelings, such as externalizing them through writing, drawing, cooking, or working out. Many children of narcissists develop other maladaptive ways of coping with trauma, such as eating disorders, substance use disorders, or obsessive-compulsive disorder (OCD), all of which are often symptoms of trauma.

Narcissistic siblings exhibit similar behaviors, and the biggest one my clients describe to me is the triangulation and one-upmanship that the narcissistic sibling portrays. They may want to be the favorite of their parents and will do things, like sabotage their siblings, to come off as the healthy child while they portray their healthy sibling as being flawed. They can even create smear campaigns against their sibling that might lead to the parent believing that the healthy child is unwell: projection on full display.

NARCISSISTIC SPOUSE OR SIGNIFICANT OTHER

While this chapter is built upon classic narcissistic behavior, there are subtleties that need to be highlighted here. When it comes to an intimate relationship, nobody falls in love faster than a narcissist who needs somewhere to live. If, on the other hand, you get swept away by a narcissist who has a place to live, they will want to move you in or even buy a new house with you, pronto! You may find them talking about this very quickly after meeting them. They will want to be on the deed and may even put it under an "LLC" to make it more difficult for you to have any access to this major asset later on. They will want to move fast for a variety of reasons, including, on the down-low, wanting to secure the constant supply that they get from having a live-in punching bag. In all relationships with narcissists, whether they are familial or not, you will find yourself walking on eggshells. If you live with the narcissistic abuser, this will continue without relief until you exist in a state of perpetual confusion.

Part of this confusion comes from the narcissist's ever-changing moods, opinions, behaviors, and mixed messages. There will be double entendres (messages delivered with two different meanings) designed to perplex, mystify, disorient, or puzzle you. They will also dole out charming and then cruel behaviors on a whim—or in a more calculated manner, depending on what they are looking to attain in a particular moment. Trying to make sense of their behavior may lead you to become extremely dazed and demoralized. These dreadful behaviors only worsen over time, and on a daily basis, the turbulence will create an upheaval in your physical, emotional, and spiritual being.

Although this is the case for anyone in a relationship with a narcissist, what makes this all the more extreme is that the narcissist's live-in partner will be the *only* person who witnesses their horrible behavior. The world sees them as the perfect parent, philanthropist, boss, neighbor, and community member. Behind closed doors, an altogether different story is unfolding. Things may seem to be humming along in a healthy way, and then a darker side of them will inevitably resurface, throwing you off-balance and starting the cycle of abuse all over again. They may apologize with the persuasiveness of a trained thespian and then, just like a professional actor who hears the word "CUT!" they will turn off the waterworks and grab a glazed doughnut from craft services. As time marches on, the version of the person you thought you loved will become less and less visible and they will be increasingly revealed as the unforgiving, remorseless, dark, and icy creature they truly are.

WARNING SIGNS THAT YOU'RE LIVING WITH A NARCISSIST

Living with a narcissist is comparable to having contractions while in labor, with the peaks increasing over time and the valleys becoming a distant memory. Keep in mind, though, that narcissists can often be charming people in public and/or in the early stages of a narcissistic abuse cycle. As such, you probably jumped into cohabitating with a suspected narcissist before you realized what they were.

Loving a narcissist is a labyrinth of blind alleys and dead-end roads. Being confused becomes normal and it becomes necessary for many to flee this scenario. According to Women Against Abuse, one of the nation's largest domestic violence advocacy and service providers, most will attempt to do so seven times before finally dislodging themselves.[1]

While I want to provide you with coping strategies, ultimately, the safest coping strategy is to make an escape plan. We will go over this in depth in Part 3, but later in this chapter, we'll discuss why it's so critical to escape. If you suspect that you are living with a narcissist, here's a list of things you might experience (or have already experienced).

You Feel Isolated

If you're living with a narcissist, you will . . .

- Slowly be made to feel bad if you have any relationships with other people, mostly of the opposite sex
- Start to hear small comments about how your narcissistic partner does not like your friends, or they may point out things about them and probe into any problems you may have had with them in the past, cultivating mistrust
- Begin to revisit old issues with friends, family, and colleagues, so as to get you to move away emotionally from others you trust
- Be berated on your return home from work or any socializing event, making you not want to repeat the mistake of acting in an autonomous way ever again

By isolating you in this way, the narcissist's goal is twofold: to get you away from your support network so that they can take all your energy, and to abuse you around fewer witnesses. They may make you feel bad for doing things with your family and accuse you of not being loving whenever you are not fully focused on them.

They Lower Your Self-Esteem

The narcissist is adept at chipping away at your confidence. They may:

- Make snide little comments about what you are eating or what you are wearing
- Be an armchair psychologist, spending countless hours instructing *you* on ways that you need to work on yourself
- Make you start to feel that you are "not good enough" or "less than"
- Make you feel that they are the best you could do in selecting a partner, based on exaggerations that they make about themselves
- Make you start to believe that they are the best for you, so you should not leave them

- Threaten to leave, themselves, as a ploy to get you to beg for them to stay, preying on the low self-esteem they've instilled in you

You Get the Silent Treatment

If you have ever had a disagreement with anyone, you may notice that you both take a break from communicating with each other. Although that can happen normally between spouses, siblings, friends, neighbors, and coworkers, the narcissist uses this as a tool with a frequency that you may ultimately recognize has a rhythm: the cycle of abuse. The narcissist views the silent treatment in a few ways. First, it is an opportunity to groom or train you to come crawling back to them, which helps them maintain their preferred power dynamic. Second, they want to keep you focused on them and sap you of your energy, so you will not be able to function in your daily life. They may do this before you have an important presentation, or on days when you have a lot going on, to literally ruin your day and have the focus stay on them in yet another energy grab.

Some staples of arguing with a narcissist include the following.

- Disagreements are often one-sided, and you may not have even done anything wrong.
- The expectation from the narcissist is that you apologize for the wrong they say you have committed, and until you "learn your lesson," they will not talk to you. Here, the silent treatment is a form of **stonewalling** and a tool to absolve themselves from all blame.
- You may feel that you are constantly being "punished" when the narcissist stops answering your calls, texts, or any other forms of communication.
- Apologies seldom happen, nor does a shared interest in reconnection and a resolution to the issue at hand. Some narcissists apologize frequently, but their actions never line up.
- Disagreements don't lead to short cooldown periods, after which you both come back at a later time to discuss what went wrong and decide how to move forward.

- They may sequester themselves in a different location, claiming to be "working," but you feel that something has changed and that they are punishing you for some unknown reason with the silent treatment, over and over again.

As humans, we enjoy being liked and appreciated by the people in our lives. As such, the silent treatment is a powerful way to create a mal-adaptive pattern and ultimately cause damage to the person being punished by it. Healthy people want to get out of this dark mind-set when they're in conflict, but for the narcissist, there is no desire to create connection, only a determination to get their own needs met and at others' expense. They will hold out until you take the blame, and they can afford to because they will utilize supplemental supplies in the interim.

They Have a Lack of Boundaries

Live-in narcissists will start to treat you as property. This will include your having very little say over *anything*. Ways that they lack or push boundaries may include the following.

- Anytime you push back against what they think should be happening, they will guilt-trip you or become angry.
- They may go through your belongings, become your business manager, or want to "share" everything, so they are better prepared to remove any boundaries or "barriers" to their being able to fully control your life.
- If you were to ask them about these activities, you might be made to feel crazy or be accused of being paranoid or jealous.
- Push through closed doors in your home
- Film you in your home
- Text you repeatedly when you are working or busy

There is a double standard at work here. Although the narcissist wants total control over your life and will encroach upon your boundaries over time until you are cornered, you should expect no input on their actions or choices in return. You might see them hide in the bathroom on their phone and wonder what they are doing. The likeliness is that they are doing something unsavory, at best.

They Seek Sexual Dominance

The narcissist not only inherently needs to always be desired, but they also will push the boundaries of sex as far as they possibly can. Many of my clients report being raped, sodomized, or forced to participate in orgies, among many other very sick and sadistic behaviors perpetrated under the coercive control of their abuser. The narcissist finds sex to be a way that they can feel something. Many narcissists do not feel much, and that is, in great part, why they cause chaos so often. They want to feel something. Sex is the supreme way for them to feel anything at all. Because of this, it becomes an obsession and they are very well devoted to getting it at all costs.

You May Be Recorded or Surveilled

The narcissist starts their smear campaign *long* before they discard you. So they are always laying the groundwork for the day that they know they will be done exploiting you.

In this vein, they may:

- Record you doing such things as reacting to their abuse, drinking, using drugs, performing sex acts, or some other behavior that they know might paint you in a bad light to your friends, family, the press, or the judicial system.
- Do small things to agitate or aggravate you, such as pinch you, pull your hair, poke you while you are sleeping, or grab your neck, so that you might become reactive. They are the ceaseless antagonist, and to live with them is to give them free rein to practice this behavior continuously.
- Have surveillance on you in the home or be stalking you. Plenty of my clients report that there are certain areas of the house where they will not go because cameras are set up there. In many cases, you may come off looking crazy because the narcissist

pushes every button when the camera is not rolling, and then only captures the part where you get pushed too far. Even if the cameras are not functioning or recording, the narcissist likes to make their victims think they are being watched so they can feel intimidated.

- Coerce their victims into sharing embarrassing or damning recordings of themselves as a pledge of loyalty. Some may even try to get you to use a racial or homophobic slur on video. They will later threaten to use this footage against you or threaten to share it with your employer or loved ones.

You Are Treated Badly During Illness or a Death in the Family

Nowhere else is it clearer that you are dealing with a narcissist than when you need care for anything from the common cold to the death of a beloved dog or family member. In these cases, the narcissist will be nowhere to be found. They do not care that you have needs. *Only their needs matter.* They also see things like this as a fracture of their fantastical thinking.

Many of my clients report that what prompted them to understand they were with a narcissist was when they were discarded after being diagnosed with cancer or another illness. The narcissist has no interest in a caregiving role . . . *at all.* The narcissist may also:

- Discount doctors' opinions
- Minimize your symptoms
- Parade others around with a similar illness, in an effort to shame their victim into believing that the sickness is a mental manifestation of their own weakness
- Play sick themselves, feigning symptoms that show they are "worse" than you, in what is clinically known as a *factitious disorder.* Factitious disorders are generally born of the need for attention and sympathy. Narcissists with a factitious disorder will

openly talk about their illness, go to appointments, and even start fund-raisers for themselves. Unlike hypochondriacs, individuals with factitious disorders, such as Munchausen's by proxy, know they/their children are not sick; they are just good liars who crave the spotlight. Most people would consider it morally repugnant to cash in on a serious illness, such as cancer, and that is why so many narcissists pull this off. Be hyper aware of someone accusing you of Munchausen's by proxy because the narcissist may be giving you information into what they may be doing to your child.

Alternatively, some narcissists will deny any illnesses and almost *never* go to the doctor or dentist, though there are certainly cases where they would play the victim. This is because they consider themselves uniquely immune to illness because any malady would put a crack in their fake and fantastical self.

They Exhibit Deviant Behaviors

When you live with a narcissist, you will see behind the curtain, where the narcissist keeps their private, most deviant behaviors. This might include:

- Partaking in illegal activities
- Drug abuse
- Lying about smoking cigarettes or doing drugs
- Lying with ease to others
- Demanding sex at all hours of the day
- Coercing you into doing things that feel taboo, "wrong," risky, or are downright painful
- Using two or more phones, claiming one is for business, even though they likely use it to communicate with other supply or sex workers. They also use them to watch pornography.
- Pacing anxiously
- Ignoring responsibilities

The narcissist engages in these deviant behaviors with impunity in your home. Because of the smear campaign they've already started against you, they feel confident that few, if any, outsiders will take your word over theirs, and they will even sometimes tell their victims, "Nobody will believe you."

They Ruin Holidays and Birthdays

Living with a narcissist during the holiday season is a marathon game of "What kind of shit are they going to come up with to torture me and appear to be the best in front of company today?" They will either lavish you with thoughtful gifts or become sullen and not want to celebrate, or both. They often take momentous occasions as an opportunity to take a nap in front of everyone, to show just how little they really care or to get you angered.

They will turn what should be a celebratory time into a time of suffering and tears. They may fish for compliments by offering up compliments to you, and when you do not deliver in kind, they will punish you with passive aggression and the silent treatment . . . *again*.

Every client I have says this rings true for them, and it certainly did for me. Narcissists make a special effort around the holidays to spread their toxicity by distorting expectations and cultural norms. They will return gifts or take issue with whatever you get them because it will not live up to their fantastical expectations; alternatively, if they appreciate your gift, they may still return it, as they may be paranoid that you, in turn, are love-bombing *them*.

Your Things Go Missing

On a truly alarming note, a narcissist may hide your car keys so that you are trapped in the home and cannot escape their abuse. What's more, many narcissists, in their preparation for the inevitable discard, will cherry-pick items from your most cherished belongings, such as money, jewelry, pictures, clothing, and artwork, to keep as "trophies" to leverage against you or to just destroy when you are parting ways. As such, you may realize after you have gotten away from them that things are missing.

In my case, my abuser poured bleach all over my clothes in the driveway as I was fleeing. This is not uncommon. Many clients have reported to me that their ex destroyed their belongings; they may even ejaculate, urinate, spit, or defecate on your belongings at the end of the relationship.

You Witness Their Paranoid Anxiety

It is hard for the narcissist to keep up with all the lies they tell, so they become increasingly anxious over time. A lot of my clients report that they think their abuser is paranoid and that they pace the yard, waiting for something to happen to them. They also have a low social conscience, so they never really get the attention they think they deserve, which creates further anxiety in them.

This place of uncertainty and ambiguity is not a place a narcissist likes to be in because any loss of control frightens them. The narcissist must protect themselves at all costs and will do whatever they can to maintain a feeling of control in their own lives. It doesn't matter what the situation is. For instance, their live-in partner's deciding what will be made for dinner could feel like a loss of control for them, therefore setting off anxiety and paranoia.

They are also scared of being exposed, so they are always on the defensive. They present as confident and competent, but this is an act. The narcissist sees danger in everything and everyone because each new experience or person they encounter has the potential to expose who they really are. This is especially the case if they are involved in criminal activities or have created foes in business. The only thing that matters is the narcissist's belief that their true selves could be found out. They never know what someone's true intention is, and they think that others may be plotting the same way they are.

They Triangulate You Against Other People

Triangulation is a relational dynamic in which two people disagree and a third person gets pulled into the disagreement; this forms a "triangle" within the argument. By bringing in a third party to agree with them, the narcissist can easily make you feel crazy. This often happens in cults, or even in the case of children of narcissistic parents, because you are totally outnumbered by those who support the narcissist's viewpoint. It serves the narcissist to make you feel outnumbered, which is exactly why they do this. Narcissists often use triangulation to:

- Distract from the real issue or argument (gaslighting)
- Tip the scales of the argument in their favor
- Reinforce their sense of superiority

It can look like your partner's bringing your friends or cohorts into an argument so that they can have these people choose their side. They might share with you that their ex won't leave them alone or wants to get back together, to get you to reassure them of your devotion or behave in certain ways that fill their narcissistic supply. They might call your mother and complain about how badly you're mistreating them, so you will be reprimanded by her. In so doing, in the hands of a narcissist, triangulation is an absolutely intentional tool of manipulation and control and they hide behind it. They also do this with attorneys in the postseparation phase, hiding behind attorney/client privilege.

You're Sleep Deprived

Narcissists will want your full attention at all hours, and they also like to torture you. This is a recipe for sleep deprivation. They may become antagonistic and pick fights with you when they know you have a big day the next day, or punish you for being tired. They may have strange sleeping habits, themselves, such as sleeping very little at night and taking naps throughout the day instead. We often make excuses for their mid–Broadway show naps with "He's tired from all of the work he is doing," or by thinking, *"I hope I can get some rest, while he's sleeping, from the constant abuse I am enduring."*

Narcissists use sleep deprivation to control you; it's all part of the manipulation, gaslighting, and mind games designed to break you down and get you into a foggier state. Many will even take you on trips or work you to the bone until your reasoning and clarity of thought are diminished. The narcissist will have you running ragged doing their bidding, and you will inevitably break down. You may notice weight loss, frequent head colds, autoimmune issues, and a variety of physical ailments. There is no shortage of data indicating that chronic stress—stress that occurs consistently over a long period of time—can have a negative impact on a person's immune system and physical health. If you are constantly under stress from living with an abuser or having to continue to engage with one, you may experience physical symptoms, such as chest pain, headaches, trouble sleeping, or high blood pressure. Other symptoms of narcissistic abuse may include upset stomach, indigestion, heartburn, and nausea.

They Manipulate the Thermostat

Many narcissists will use the thermostat in a car or home to make you feel too hot or too cold, to create an uncomfortable environment where they can gauge how much you will tolerate. This "turning up and down of the dial" is a tremendous metaphor for what they will do throughout the relationship, always measuring what you will endure.

They Restrict Your Eating or Force You to Eat

As mentioned earlier, a tactic for the narcissist or cult leader is to control your eating habits. They may even get you on the scale to weigh you and frame it as an act of "love." They want to ensure you are caring for yourself. Yeah. Sure.

When the narcissist is restricting your caloric intake, they are micromanaging one of the most personal and private parts of a human experience. Talk about a boundary violation! Many of them hoard food as a way to one-up others and diligently keep track of every item in the refrigerator and pantry. Many don't like to share food, not even with their own children. The very same narcissist may make you feel bad for eating one day, and make you feel bad for not eating the next.

When we eat, we are prioritizing ourselves, which is automatically a trigger for the narcissist. Narcissists don't want their partners and family members to act with self-love. Self-love promotes feelings of importance and independence, which threaten the narcissist's autocratic rule. Controlling and scrupulously accounting for the resources essential to our very survival is one of the ways narcissists flex in the relationship. Perhaps the most disturbing examples of food used as a weapon to manipulate and control come from the children of narcissistic parents. Many narcissistic parents invent arbitrary rules that govern when their child can and can't eat, without any regard for or concern about the child's needs. They may shame their children for their appearance if they are "too thin" or "too heavy," and may even put a padlock on the refrigerator door, the pantry, or the liquor cabinet.

You Must Focus on Their Happiness

The narcissistic partner cannot compete with anyone else, even their own children when it comes to getting your attention. When you move in with them, this gets worse because they will monopolize your time, requiring you to do all the household chores while also being ready to go out or entertain, in spite of how tired you become. Many people who are with narcissists have pets with them, and the narcissist actually likes pets because they get supply from animals. However, keep in mind that if you become your dog's "person," this will upset the narcissistic abuser. If you are giving your own children or pets attention, this will trigger them, and they will try to fracture those relationships, often by any means necessary.

You Lose Yourself

Ultimately, there is no way to live with a narcissist and not lose yourself. Your life becomes all about them, and the dreams and goals you once had will slowly disappear as control shifts from you to the narcissist. As your friends disappear and your career starts to fall apart, you may wake up one day and realize that you sacrificed everything for a fake person who ultimately discards you. It is a slow burn that over time robs you of all the things that make you special. Most of my clients report it happening so gradually that it was nearly undetectable.

WHY IT CAN BE DIFFICULT TO BREAK AWAY

At its core, living with a narcissist is to live in constant turmoil, and you may be the only person who sees it. When you try to tell anyone what is happening at home, they may say things like "But that's your mom" or "But he definitely loves you." This can compound your turmoil tremendously.

Many therapists not trained in narcissistic personality disorder may also compound the issue by trying to have the "There's two sides to the story" perspective, which, again, does nothing to help those people suffering at the hands of an abuser. In the end, because they have been so manipulative for so long, narcissists will even gaslight the judicial system into believing *you* are the problem.

If you are reading this book as the loved one of a suspected victim of narcissistic abuse, never downplay what they are experiencing. I cannot tell you how many people and friends I thought loved me sided with my abuser and made me feel that I was the problem. It was truly devastating to me. I liken the first, initial discard as an earthquake and the loss of friends afterward as aftershocks or tremors. I am so thankful to also have had people who believed me.

This Jekyll and Hyde experience is what makes it so hard to process narcissistic abuse for yourself, so how could you even expect others to understand it? You may even wonder at times whether your abuser has multiple personalities because you will see profoundly different versions of the same person. There is the loving partner you fell for who shows up in public, and then there is the person who sabotages you, devalues you, and feels utter rage toward you in private. It can sometimes even feel as if each personality doesn't know the other one exists. Narcissists do not have different personalities. They know what they are doing.

It is dangerous work to dance with the devil, so to live with one is a game of life and death. Ironically, living with a narcissist is not living with a narcissist; living with a narcissist is *dying* with a narcissist.

They may convince you that people are "jealous of us" and you are a "power couple" that needs to be isolated from others for your own protection.

WHY IT'S SO DAMAGING TO STAY

Anyone who has ever lived with a narcissist has had to deal with gaslighting and circular conversations. This is also referred to as "word salad" and will break down your ability to discern fact from fiction. It will confuse you so much that you may even end up with a brain injury. There is now data indicating that not only do the people who are in an intimate relationship with a narcissist develop a brain injury as a result of their abuse but also the children of narcissists are left with brain damage from their narcissistic parent.[2] When children suffer at the hands of a narcissistic abuser, crucial brain regions are affected, including the hippocampus and amygdala. These changes lead to devastating effects on the lives of their victims.

The *hippocampus* is a paired structure tucked inside each temporal lobe. It helps store and release memory. The hippocampus is especially vital to short-term memory, the way the mind retains a piece of data for a few moments, after which it either gets transferred to permanent memory or is immediately forgotten. According to psychologist and *New York Times* science journalist Daniel Goleman's 2006 book *Social Intelligence*, everything we learn, everything we read, everything we do, everything we understand, and everything we experience counts on the hippocampus to function correctly.[3] Learning is therefore dependent on short-term memory, which means that the education of children of narcissistic parents may be adversely impacted by their abuse. The continual retention of memories demands a large amount of neuronal activity, and the brain's production of and connections to new neurons take place in the hippocampus.

Goleman also states, in *Social Intelligence*, that the hippocampus is especially vulnerable to ongoing emotional distress because of the damaging effects of cortisol. When the body endures ongoing stress, cortisol affects the rate at which neurons are either added or subtracted from the hippocampus. When the neurons are attacked by cortisol, the hippocampus loses neurons and is reduced in size.[4] In a study conducted by a team at the University of New Orleans and Stanford University, researchers discovered that patients with the highest baseline of the stress hormone cortisol and a greater number of trauma symptoms had the greatest decreases in hippocampal volume over time.[5] In other words, the longer you stay with an emotionally abusive person, the more deterioration you can expect of your hippocampus. This neurological process may enhance feelings of confusion, cognitive dissonance, and abuse amnesia in victims of narcissistic abuse.

The *amygdala*, meanwhile, is where such emotions as fear, guilt, envy, and shame are born. Goleman, in *Social Intelligence*, explains that cortisol stimulates the amygdala, whereas it impairs the hippocampus, forcing our attention onto the emotions we feel while restricting our ability to take in new information.[6] The amygdala is also responsible for the fight-or-flight response. Victims of narcissistic abuse live in this state almost daily, and over time we remember the things we felt, saw, and heard, each time we have a painful experience. These are called flashbacks or, as I sometimes call them, the "reeling feeling," where it feels as if you are watching a movie reel of what happened in the relationship. Subliminal triggers for such stressful events, such as seeing photos of a certain person or place, or hearing a certain song, will set off an intense emotion or reaction.

Even after the toxic relationship has ended, victims of narcissistic abuse suffer trauma, panic attacks, phobias, depression, anxiety, substance abuse, self-harm, eating disorders, unwanted pregnancies, autoimmune disorders, miscarriages, suicide attempts, sleep disorders, and gastrointestinal conditions, but the most prevalent complaint I get from my clients is the trauma to their brain, due to the triggering of their primal fears by their overactive amygdala.

Again, *narcissistic abuse literally changes the brain*. In fact, *duration of stress is almost as destructive as acute stress*. In other words, the prolonged abuse a victim experiences from the narcissist is at least as treacherous as a direct punch to the face.

There is hope, though, to repair the damaged brain, and fortunately, as brain scans have now shown—thanks to the magic of neuroplasticity and, in many ways, the work of Bessel van der Kolk, author of *The Body Keeps the Score*,[7] and his team—it is possible for the hippocampus to regrow. An effective method is the use of eye movement desensitization and reprocessing (EMDR) therapy. EMDR is simply described as therapist-directed lateral eye movements and a variety of other stimuli, including hand-tapping and audio stimulation. In a clinical setting, for instance, a trained therapist may prompt you to move your eyes back and forth while they work through a verbal prompt with you. One recent study showed that eight to twelve sessions of EMDR for patients with trauma showed an average 6 percent increase in the volume of their hippocampus. EMDR also helps counteract the hyperarousal of the amygdala, allowing the brain to more appropriately direct what needs to happen instead of remaining unnecessarily triggered by problematic emotions.[8]

There is also a lot of data coming out now on alternative treatments for trauma, including psychedelics. I recently attended the Psychotherapy Networker Symposium in Washington, DC, at which van der Kolk highlighted some of the ways that people are benefiting from new and alternative treatments for brain trauma, including MDMA (3, 4-methylenedioxymethamphetamine, commonly known as ecstasy or Molly). Somatic therapy practices, as well as reparenting or identifying your separate "parts" through imagery, can add tremendous value to recovery.

Leaving is incredibly difficult but necessary to fully heal. It is extremely important to get in front of a therapist who understands narcissistic abuse to get help and develop a safety plan. An organization like mine, Tell A Therapist, INC., can refer you to a narcissistic abuse–savvy therapist in your state. You may feel that you are all alone, an emotion the narcissist wants you to feel, but there are millions of people who have experienced this abuse who are here to help. I honor the reasons many stay with a narcissist, but I still feel strongly that it is better for your overall well-being to leave, *especially* in the case of children of narcissists. They could be groomed so that they grow up to harm others by doing their toxic parent's bidding, or they may have trauma themselves from living with a narcissist. One way that some of my clients try to get away from their narcissistic parents is to try to see them only on holidays if that is a possibility. The idea here is to practice harm reduction and minimize exposure as much as you can; go low contact.

When you live with a narcissist, traumatic brain injury is not a risk, it is an imminent threat. Being able to say I survived is something I do not take for granted. Many do not survive living with a narcissist, even if it is the death of their soul.

You *can* recover, though, and live a better life than before, because your new normal is filled with "god winks," synchronicities, and silver linings in abundance. You need only look for them. They are there.

THERAPY TIP: FIVE SENSES

I want to bring your attention back to our conversation about physical, mental, and emotional safety, both before and after you leave a narcissistically abusive situation.

It is also important to your safety to make sure that you are able to self-soothe in the event that you are still dealing with a narcissist.

In dialectical behavioral therapy (DBT), to soothe ourselves, we go to the five senses if we are feeling triggered, destabilized, anxious, panicked, or if we need to feel grounded. Taking a moment to pause and focus on external stimuli can help us feel grounded and calmer.

Sense of Sight

- Find pictures of places or things that you find soothing to look at. The pictures can be of different cities, natural landscapes, or artistic still-lifes.
- Go to a museum or a gallery.
- Watch a movie that is famous for its beautiful cinematography. Make sure that it is a story that won't be difficult for you to watch.

Sense of Hearing

- Talk to a person whose voice makes you happy or you enjoy hearing.
- Listen to music. You want to stay as close to your "baseline" as you can, so no music that is too frantic and nothing that is too depressing. I like to listen to something with no lyrics, such as jazz music. (Benny Goodman is my favorite.)
- Go outside and enjoy the liveliness of the sounds around you (e.g., birds, wind, people chattering).
- If you play a musical instrument or sing in your free time, taking some time to practice a favorite song may help soothe you.

- Listen to an audiobook or a podcast that you enjoy.

Sense of Smell

- Wear a perfume or cologne that you enjoy the smell of.
- Light a scented candle or use an essential oil diffuser.
- Cook a meal that smells delicious to you.
- Buy some scented flowers or indoor plants.
- Hug a person whose smell makes you feel calm.
- Go someplace where you enjoy the scent (e.g., a flower shop, perfume shop, restaurant, bakery).

Sense of Taste

- Cook your favorite meal; eat it slowly and savor its taste.
- Go to your favorite restaurant and order your favorite meal.
- Enjoy your favorite snacks or comfort food.
- Make yourself a cup of coffee, tea, cocoa, or anything else that you enjoy drinking.
- Eat a piece of fresh fruit.
- Chew gum or eat some sweets. A study done by the National Library of Medicine indicates chewing gum can reduce stress.[9]

Sense of Touch

- Take a soft blanket and wrap yourself in it.
- Pet an animal. This is my go-to for touch, and it checks a couple of boxes (e.g., soft touch, pleasant scent, happy visual).
- Wear comfortable clothes and enjoy how they feel on your skin.
- Take a shower or a bubble bath, at whatever temperature you find most soothing.
- Get a massage, or practice a self-massage, such as kneading the soles of your feet.
- Touch something smooth, velvety, or fluffy.

Chapter 7

Why We Fall for
the Narcissist

*When Carrie-Ann met Mason, he was so attentive and he seemed
to know everyone. She admitted that she loved being treated like
a queen, and their relationship was fast and furious. When Mason
started to change, she couldn't believe it. "I was just . . . it just didn't
make sense," she told me during a session. "It was like whiplash.
And, look, the sex was fantastic. I guess I just couldn't believe that
someone who I had such an intense connection with could be such
a monster."*

———— ⊗ ————

Most people are seeking connection, friendship, passion, intimacy,
true love, safety, and security when they look for an intimate
partner. This is similar to what people seek in a religious organization
that may be legitimate, or a cult. The benefits of having a healthy social
life and connection with others are completely backed by science. Social

connections influence our long-term health in ways every bit as powerful as adequate sleep, a good diet, and not smoking. An abundance of studies have shown that people who have satisfying relationships with family, friends, and their community are happier, have fewer health problems, and live longer.

The quality of our relationships matter. For example, one study found that middle-aged women in a highly satisfying marriage or long-term partnership have a lower risk of cardiovascular disease compared with those in a less-satisfying marriage.[1]

Conversely, a relative lack of social ties is associated with depression and cognitive decline later in life, as well as with increased mortality. One study by Harvard Medical School, which examined data from more than 309,000 people, found that a lack of strong relationships increased a person's risk of premature death from all causes by 50 percent—an effect on mortality risk that is not only roughly comparable to smoking up to fifteen cigarettes a day, but also greater than that of obesity and physical inactivity.[2] There is no shortage of data telling us that connection with other humans is healthy and that we are innately and organically a social species.

That being said, we don't often realize who we might be partnering up with and the level of damage they may be capable of causing. Many of us have the best intentions and are seeking a true connection, but ultimately get stuck in a mess with a chameleon who blends into whatever they learn about what you want to see. What makes us fall for them? Why and how did this happen? How could we have missed the signs? How did we become sucked into this vortex? The quick answer is that nothing the narcissist says or does is what it seems, and they are a master manipulator.[3] They will be savvy at reeling you in through a variety of methods, and unless you really understand this disorder and the red flags, you may miss it. If your boundaries are not strong and you are not sturdy in your independent thought process, you can fall for one too. We all can. The diversity of the victims in my practice run the gamut, but one thing is clear: we just didn't know.

And it's not our fault.

DON'T JUDGE A BOOK BY ITS COVER.

Narcissists exude self-confidence and will go to great lengths to convince you that they are your perfect mate, putting on a show to capture your heart. Your initial interaction with a narcissist may even seem like a "coincidence," though this is only because they may have been stalking you and they will make it seem as though fate were involved.

Researcher Mitja Back and his colleagues conducted studies to figure out why a narcissist makes such a great first impression. Along with his colleague Michael Dufner, Dr. Back sent male participants into the streets of a German city with the task of approaching twenty-five random women and getting their contact information. Research assistants followed the men and then interviewed the women they'd approached, asking whether they'd liked the man and if they were attracted to him. The more narcissistic the man was, the more contacts he made, and the more appealing he seemed to women.[4]

One of the main reasons, Dr. Back discovered, was that the narcissist's self-representation and their ability to be amazing salespeople and actors cements this narrative: They focus on presentation, including their clothes, grooming, perfume or cologne, their car, and accessories. Some may be physically attractive, but all of them work at maintaining a polished and appealing look. Many will not leave the house without a full face of makeup or a three-piece suit. It's like putting on their uniform—the narcissistic cloak of bullshit. They will captivate others with their reflective listening or responding to those persons by reflecting back what they heard (keep in mind that they are collecting data), a great sense of humor, a sexy smirk or smile, amazing manners, and a ton of compliments.

While the narcissist's performance appears to be directed at the person they are with, it's really not about the victim. It's all about validating the narcissistic person; external validation is what keeps the narcissist's false self alive.

Narcissists know that they only exist when other people acknowledge them. They use people as a mirror to reflect themselves back to them, and this can very quickly create an "out of sight, out of mind" situation in which, if you leave the narcissist alone for any amount of time, they will grow bitter, angry, and sometimes violent so as to keep your attention. They will seek supply almost instantaneously elsewhere. Because they don't have a true sense of self, they're constantly assessing people's reactions and opinions to get a sense of who they are and what they're worth. These external sources regulate their self-esteem, and so they will constantly calculate ways to get supply as if their life depended on it.

Narcissists are obsessed with appearance and care deeply about looks, money, and the perception of status, so it should come as no surprise that they would wield these characteristics as a way to entice others. Some are supereasy to spot, whereas some of the more benign, vulnerable, or covert narcissists are not. **They lack depth and the ability to connect, emotionally, through communication, so they may use sarcasm or passive aggression as a way to devalue you, but you may not see this at first.**

Sarcasm is a shame-based communication that is kind of like passive aggression's older brother. It comes easily to the narcissist, so be careful around people who pride themselves on sarcastic and snarky humor. They use these tools to make themselves feel better but will wrap veiled insults and punishments in a "humorous" bow.

THE NARCISSIST IS AN EXPERT AT SWINDLING.

Studies show that narcissists need relationships yet tend to scout for the next connection that suits their needs while they're still in a relationship. As a result, it's highly possible that they will cheat on their current romantic partner. In other words, they are in a constant phase of transferability. They will be thinking about the next victim long before they discard anyone.

This inability to be satiated is a root cause for why they can never be happy and content in a relationship; they are always playing their games of manipulation and lies with this supply, past supplies (in their **hoovering** phases), and the next supply (putting out feelers for what's ahead) at the same time. I often think of this as a train, with the most recent supply being the caboose *until* they add a new car onto the line. They will also take the knowledge they gain from each supply and use it to punish past supplies. If you tell a narcissist that you have always wanted to go to Ibiza, they will not take you there, but they will take the next supply there just to rub it in your face on social media. Is this punishment for something you did? Nope; it's just their vindictive thought patterns.

They may also steal from one supply and give to the next. The "Tinder Swindler," a man named Shimon Hayut, traveled around Europe, presenting himself as the son of Russian-Israeli diamond mogul Lev Leviev. He used the dating app Tinder to contact women as Simon Leviev and tricked them into lending him money that he would never repay, but that he would use to seduce the next supply. **This is their game—that of the professional con person.** Some of my clients have reported that after they became engaged, the narcissist swapped out their engagement stone for glass and they had no idea. They may buy you fake jewelry and let you believe these items are authentic as well.

THEY ARE OFTEN GOOD LOVERS.

Narcissists like sex, and they are very focused on how well they perform—alas, it's not for you, but for them. Sex with a narcissist can be confusing because this may seem like a real and positive bonding experience, but it is nothing more than an active representation of two narcissistic traits: entitlement and exploitation.

YOU MAY HAVE BEEN RAISED BY A NARCISSISTIC PERSON.

If you were raised or surrounded by narcissists growing up, your odds of dating a narcissist are higher. This is because you may have been robbed of your identity early on by the narcissistic parent who groomed you to be someone who lives in subjugation, thereby making you familiar with and even comfortable in these environments. Being around a narcissist becomes normalized.

Some children of narcissists may even have narcissistic characteristics themselves. A good example of this would be a child growing up in a family that uses passive aggression almost as their exclusive "language." This child may learn later in life how to communicate in a healthy manner, but it is something they would never have learned in the narcissistic home.

All of these can further "normalize" being in relationships with a narcissist; the adult child's compass is broken.

Some children may make decisions and choices based on how much they want their parents to be proud of them. Later in life, this can transform into making choices based on how happy their partner will be with them, so they may become dependent on the other person to make them happy and validate their self-worth.

Some children may have a sick parent that they were always trying to "fix" or make happy. This prompts them to want to do the same in their adult intimate relationships, giving up their lives to their parents and then their partners through servitude. They will be overly accommodating of other people in their lives and have few boundaries. They may feel that they can never say no to anything that their partner wants them to do.

YOU MIGHT BE CODEPENDENT.

Codependency is a learned behavior that affects an individual's ability to have a healthy, mutually satisfying relationship. It is a dysfunctional relationship dynamic in which one person assumes the role of "the giver," sacrificing their own needs and well-being for the sake of the other, "the taker." The bond in question doesn't have to be romantic; it can occur just as easily between parent and child, friends, and family members. Codependency is important to understand because a lot of victims are brought up to be this way and will find themselves more prone to being in an abusive relationship.

The term "codependency" first appeared in substance abuse circles to describe a lopsided relationship that has been consumed and controlled by one person's addiction. It grew in popularity and became shorthand for any enabling relationship, and, given how we've established that narcissism is an addiction to attention, it is little surprise that it is often discussed in narcissistic abuse recovery. Codependency is not a clinical diagnosis or a personality disorder, but it does highlight some of the ways people can find themselves entangled with a toxic person.

YOU MAY BE BLINDED BY THE LIFESTYLE.

Narcissists are often engaged in fun activities, so it is easy to get caught up in the things they are involved in, such as concerts, golfing, the country club, the plastic surgeon's office, vacations, the gym, the salon, or night-clubs. They *love* pageantry and posturing, and they tend to really love to go to places where they think they may run into famous or successful people, to potentially leech off those with status.

Their natural habitat is the one in which the most people could become hypnotized by them. For instance, a narcissist may brag about being con-nected to a certain band, saying they have free front-row tickets to a show (and you end up sitting in the nosebleeds).

Many narcissists have political roles, judicial careers, and law enforce-ment gigs; they are often CEOs and powerful people, so the potential for you to have a larger-than-life experience with them—one of worldliness and expansive sophistication—can be incredibly compelling.

YOU MAY BE IMPACTED BY THE PATRIARCHY.

Narcissistic abuse victims often have an optimism about people's capacity for change. They may have a canny ability to assume others are like them; may overdisclose personal information; may be overly sociable, coopera-tive, sentimental, and honest; and may even have a "helping career," such as nurse or therapist. Many are not taught to recognize patterns of male violence, and some may even romanticize it.

For generations, Disney movies have made us want to believe in the person that is too good to be true. This creates false hope and unreal-istic expectations, given the Prince Charming bullshit being fed to us extremely early on. The patriarchy's impact on letting narcissistic abuse fly under the radar is the old "he pulled your hair, so he must like you" way of thinking. It's the demand to "kiss Grandpa hello" in spite of the child's not wanting to. In such cases, the child's bodily autonomy is taken away, and independent thinking goes right with it, especially in certain sections of society.

We do not encourage our children to color outside the lines, and this basically hands them over to abusive scenarios because they become followers. The truth is, we have been fed narratives that are harmful for far too long, and we have a systemic patriarchal issue with the way we treat females. Society as a whole is primed to be controlled by the media and organized religion, but girls/women are *superprimed* to be controlled by the impossible expectations that we put on them and the ways in which we treat them when they can't live up to the challenge: Be tough, but not too tough, or you'll be called a bitch. Be beautiful, but not too beautiful, or you'll be called vain. Be sexy, but not too sexy, or you'll be called a slut.

These mixed messages don't do anything to help women reach their truest potential, but worse than that, they can leave them confused and afraid to push past barriers. As such, they may remain underdeveloped personally, or they may adopt a role that they think society will more readily accept—at its most patriarchal extreme, this might mean "barefoot and pregnant in the kitchen."

Structural problems associated with the patriarchy undermine advocacy for gender fairness, and so when it comes to narcissistic abuse, women are set up to fail and fall into the hands of controlling people. After all, standing up for yourself isn't considered feminine! Excluding women from collective resources certainly paves the way for male domination, but moreover, we are given these subtle messages so early on that we often don't realize that a level of gender supremacy is instituted against women. We are seeing this front and center in the political arena as reproductive rights are being stripped away with the overturning of *Roe v. Wade*.

Gender prejudices are embedded in our culture, and traditional practices allocate undue privileges, recognition, resources, and power to men. This imbalance of power continues to put women at a tremendous disadvantage and a tremendous risk.

YOU MAY HAVE BEEN IMPACTED BY RELIGION.

While many of us take comfort in our spiritual beliefs, there are some basic issues and questions that confront people raised in religions that teach their believers to follow blindly the god or deity. Many of the teachings can be roadblocks to a person's self-determination.

Many religions support a faith in something "bigger" than the individual, and the individual is to do what they are told to do in the name of their god. This sentiment is so damaging to so many people who are not taught to question authority or people in positions of power.

Either by its silence or its instruction, many a church, mosque, or synagogue has communicated to the masses (specifically women) that they should stay in abusive relationships, try to be better wives, and "forgive and forget." To batterers, it has communicated that their efforts to control their wives or girlfriends are justified because women are to be subject to men in all ways and things. They have been permitted to "discipline" their wives and their children, all for the "good of the family." Christian history is filled with examples of church leaders justifying the abuse of women by men.

Cult leaders and narcissists sometimes exploit servitude to a god, paving the way to spiritual abuse; regardless of that, some religions, by their own fundamental nature, send a message to followers to forgive, love, and serve *no matter what*.

―――∞∞∞―――

Narcissists are all wolves in sheep's clothing, sweeping you off your feet with a luxurious lifestyle, charming personality, or more. I wanted to share this content so that you know you are not alone, you are not a fool or stupid, and that it's not your fault. The important thing to keep in mind is that you've realized the con, and that there is time to free yourself. You are a survivor, and you are in good company. That's what really matters.

THERAPY TIP: MEDITATION

While you may think, *"Meditation is hard; it's not for me,"* meditation can go a long way toward resolving brain trauma and injury perpetrated by narcissistic abusers. Here are some simple ways you can practice meditation on your own, whenever you choose:

- **Breathe deeply.** Developed by Edna Foa, PhD, an authority on exposure therapy for trauma, this technique is good for beginners because breathing is a natural function.
- **Focus on your exhale.**
  Breathe in through your nose and out through your mouth. Slow your breathing down, considerably.
  On exhaling, silently say to yourself, CALM or RELAX in a slow way. Example: c-a-a-a-a-a-l-m or r-e-e-e-e-e-l-a-x.
  Count slowly to 4 and then take the next inhalation.
  Practice this exercise several times a day, for 10 minutes each time.
- **Focus on the tense parts of your body.**
  Start in a comfortable, seated, relaxed position.
  Unclench your jaw, release your brow, and lower your shoulders.
- **Repeat a mantra.** This is the most important part. You can create your own mantra, such as a simple "I deserve to love myself and be loved by others" or "I am safe."

Part II

The Playbook

Whenever I meet a new client, we talk about the possibility of their having endured narcissistic abuse. To do this, we go through everything they have experienced at the hands of a possible narcissist. What has become evident as a result of this exercise is the way narcissists do so many of the same things to their victims. They all share a common modus operandi (MO).

In this part of the book, I hope to clarify the ways in which the narcissist recruits, toys with, and then pushes aside their victims—ways that express the chilling forethought that goes into their cyclical madness. I believe learning that they perform the same behaviors over and over with different supplies can be equal parts horrifying and validating. It is horrifying because you realize that they do this to person after person; it is validating because you come to learn that such actions cannot be personalized—they do not even see or care at all about the people they are harming. It wasn't your fault that they chose you.

These chapters are dedicated to the phases of the narcissist's behavior: the luring phase, the initial stalking that the narcissist practices to find a new victim; the love-bombing phase, when they pull out all stops to hook you and get you to fall for them; after this phase, the narcissist will begin to tire of their new victim, and subsequently, the discard phase shows up; lastly, the smear campaign rears its ugly head, building on the work the narcissist has done *early* on. These phases culminate in the cycle of abuse that will repeat itself over and over.

Chapter 8

"What a Coincidence!"— The Luring Phase

When Lynne first met Pat, she couldn't believe the coincidences early in their relationship: "I would go to my Starbucks and he would be there—it was this amazing synchronicity. He started showing up other places I go too." Then, he eventually showed up at her door. "I remember thinking that it was so nice, you know, that he would take that sort of time, to find out where I live and bring me flowers. And then it turned out that he loved the Tornadoes [their local baseball team] too. It seemed like fate."

⟡⟡⟡

The very first thing that a narcissist does is lie to you.

In the **luring** phase, they are meeting you under the guise of something that is altogether untrue. The narcissist may seem to show up randomly at a location you frequent—for instance, a bar or coffee shop—or may pretend that they want to use services that you provide, such as life coaching or real estate. There may be many "coincidences" in how you met, and the narcissist may tell the story of how you met, to others, over and over, as if it were some kind of divine experience or message from the universe, thereby perpetuating their narrative that you are "soulmates."

Once you've met, you may be inundated with texts, emails, and phone calls, and/or frequent deliveries of gifts, cards, and flowers. They will act like Prince or Princess Charming and portray a version of themselves that is not real. Your supposed "meet-cute" comes off as a special encounter, but this is a predator stalking their prey. They will prey on a supply's vulnerabilities and fake having interests similar to theirs, so as to reel in their latest victim.

The narcissist's tools to hook a new supply are varied, but the use of surveillance and social media are common. They may even curate pornographic pictures, cars, Rolexes, and other things to catfish (use a false identity) on various dating apps or social media platforms. The following is an in-depth look at some of the narcissist's most common luring tactics.

CYBERSTALKING/CYBER-GASLIGHTING

Cyberstalking often falls into four main types: *vindictive cyberstalking*, which involves threats; *composed cyberstalking*, which involves annoyance and harassment; *intimate cyberstalking*, which involves a person's ex or a person infatuated with their victim; and *collective cyberstalking*, in which a person is targeted by a group of individuals.

Ways that the narcissist may cyberstalk their supply include sending too many texts, emails, or messages; combing obsessively over your social media profiles; and installing cameras at your place of residence. In some cases, such as the installation of security cameras, you may see these forms of surveillance—and even think they're there to protect you—whereas in others, if the camera is hidden, you may not. They may also use spyware to monitor your behavior online or hire private investigators to do their dirty work. The more slippery narcissist may even hire people to do it so that it cannot get traced back to them.

Most people would feel intimidated and anxious if someone knew their every move, but many victims in the initial stages of the narcissistic relationship may mistake this for caring or loving behavior. They may even think that their partner can "read their mind." They may convince themselves that this is the universe making sure that their soulmate is close to them at all times, or that the coincidences they're noticing are cosmic or magical in nature. The narcissist may show up at your hairdresser's and pretend they were in the neighborhood, and you may think that they really love you or it was destiny. It is no coincidence that they keep "bumping into you."

The narcissist may *cyber-gaslight* you, which is when they hack your phone and confuse you by texting themselves from your phone number. Reading messages you don't remember sending (and, in reality, *didn't* send) can make you feel unstable and confused. The narcissist may send you content that is inappropriate or disturbing, which can leave you feeling fearful, distressed, anxious, and worried. They do strange and peculiar things to occupy your energy and have you question reality. They may hack your music playlist and then sing the songs you are listening to in the kitchen, and when you express your concern to other family members, they may accuse you of hearing or seeing things.

Cyberstalking is a growing problem. According to the Pew Research Center, 4 in 10 Americans have experienced online harassment, and 55 percent of them consider it a significant issue.[1] Cyber- and social media–based manipulation starts early and continues throughout the narcissistic relationship. These interactions do not end even if you express your displeasure or ask the narcissist to stop, in fact they may increase.

You may be experiencing cyberstalking if someone is sending you inappropriate messages or too many messages of any kind, liking all your old social media posts, manipulating you into interacting with them online, or trolling you. Impersonating someone else and sending threatening messages are also behaviors associated with narcissistic abuse online. Other ways that the narcissist may cyberstalk their target include:

- Joining the same groups and forums as you
- Commenting on or liking everything you post online
- Creating fake accounts (a.k.a. catfishing) to follow you on social media
- Messaging you repeatedly
- Hacking into or hijacking your online accounts/websites
- Attempting to extort cybersex or explicit photos from you
- Sending unwanted gifts or items to you
- Releasing your confidential information online (a.k.a. doxing), including real or fake photos of you
- Bombarding you with sexually explicit photos of themselves
- Signing you up for telemarketing scams/spam emails
- Creating fake posts designed to shame you
- Tracking your online movements through the use of external devices or malware
- Hacking into your camera on your laptop or smartphone as a way to secretly record you
- Spoof texting or calling you from phantom numbers
- Hiring private investigators to stalk you
- Continuing the harassing behavior even after being asked to stop

As in the offline world, cyberstalking has the potential to cause a wide and tragic range of physical and emotional symptoms in those who are targeted.

How to Protect Yourself: Ways you can try to protect yourself from cyberstalking include changing your passwords frequently, logging out of platforms every time you use them, never leaving your phone unattended, only using secure Wi-Fi networks, and only accepting friend requests from people you can confirm are really who they say they are.

An important note: One of the biggest things that my clients regret is deleting or destroying *anything* the narcissist sent them in conjunction with their cyberstalking and/or cyber-gaslighting. The narcissist is saving everything to use against you later, so you must keep, track, and chronicle *everything* they send you. Never toss out paperwork or have a "burn party" to extinguish old copies of anything; don't even delete horrible photos or chat threads from your phone. I know it is tempting to celebrate and rid yourself of this toxic story, but there can be serious repercussions to destroying receipts when it comes to narcissistic abuse. You will need to have proof of their behavior.

Notify your local police department if you are feeling violated online or in person. The resulting police report acts as a paper trail that you can fall back on, even if it is kept by the police station and nobody else becomes aware of it. Narcissists are adept at creating a paper trail, so it would be beneficial for you to become adept at it too.

There are no strong cyberstalking laws as of yet, but keeping a record of things that happen online that are similar to extortion can be helpful. A person may be charged with extortion if they publish or threaten to publish private photos or videos of another person with the intention of forcing them to do something they don't want to do, especially if they have communicated through interstate commerce channels, such as phones, computers, or the internet.

MIRRORING

Once the narcissist hooks you, they will learn all about your experiences, likes, dislikes, and mannerisms so as to become your own personal, twisted chameleon.

If you have ever been a new person in a group, you may have felt a little out of the loop at first. On the outside looking in, you may have noticed that the other group members are on the same wavelength, often referring to shared inside jokes and collective humor styles. They may speak in similar tones or with the same mannerisms. Some people may even begin to adopt others' accents, slang, or figures of speech.

These are examples of healthy mirroring. We all adapt the behaviors in our social systems in a variety of different ways, and some psychologists have even argued that when children do not get healthy mirroring from their parents, it can trigger pathological disorders. However, the narcissist purposely fakes a new version of themselves for each of their supplies as a way of manipulating their victim. This is extremely present in the initial phases of the narcissistic relationship and will ultimately be weaponized against you.

Normal mirroring happens organically, slowly, and with all parties' consent. The narcissist, meanwhile, fast-tracks this normal function by doing such things as copying your mannerisms—how you walk or the way you speak with your hands; learning your native language; claiming to like things you like; and adopting your hobbies, then wrapping it all in a bow of "coincidence." If you love jazz music, they love jazz music; if you love Mexican food, what do you know? They do too! They may start to dress like you or eat the same foods you do. They may even use outright lies. If you tell them that you grew up going to a certain locale, they will tell you they did as well. Your family is from a certain region of a foreign country? SAME!

Their aim here is to make you believe that you are in the company of someone who has "known you for years." It makes you feel seen and as if they really "get" you. They will study you and burn the midnight oil to figure out your vulnerabilities and passions.

Keep in mind that they will go *extremely far* with these delusional and manufactured versions of themselves. This goes far beyond Mexican food and jazz music. If you like going to the gym, gardening, chocolaty desserts, and helping at the local domestic violence shelter, so do they! If you have tattoos, suddenly they will show up with one too. Many will actually brand their victims or get a matching tattoo as a part of the mirroring.

When everything you like and value is being validated by a seemingly confident and successful person, it is easy to fall for their trap. This is all a trick to make you lower your guard. If you are not aware of what is happening, you may reveal deep and personal things about yourself to the very person that will exploit them to severely damage your life and self-worth.

Once the initial phase of the relationship has dwindled, the put-downs and devaluations start, and the dark version of mirroring begins. Now, the narcissist's mirroring switches from a positive reflection of the things you desire and value to a negative one of the things you revile and fear.

Let's say you reveal that you are worried you may turn out to be like your mother. The narcissist will store this information for use at a later date. Then, at the right moment, they'll mirror that back: "That sounds like something your mother would say." They bank this information and use it whenever they need to feel better about themselves, especially at your expense or to win an argument.

If you reveal insecurities about work, they may remind you of this by mirroring them back to you: "Are you sure you want that promotion? That sounds like it might be too much work for you. Are you really ready for that?"

Life with a narcissist is like being in a fun house without the fun: narcissistic mirroring and projection meet you at every turn. At first, you may feel dazzled, seduced by what the narcissist is showing you about yourself and about them, but before long, you feel trapped in a maze of grotesque distortions with no apparent exit.

WHY WE FALL FOR NARCISSISTIC LURING

It is an overgeneralization that narcissists have a type; their dynamic is to gain control in relationships, so they find partners with specific personality traits that can ensure their luring tactics will be successful. While not all victims may share these traits, and the narcissist will draw a supply of attention from any creature, here are some characteristics, both positive and negative, that the narcissist is able to easily manipulate in their intended victim.

- Quick to forgive
- Unhealed trauma and shame
- Highly empathetic
- Unwavering loyalty
- Low self-esteem
- Overly accommodating
- Strong accountability/overly responsible

We've discussed the luring *phase* of the narcissistic relationship here, but make no mistake: luring behaviors cycle through again in the narcissistic cycle of abuse. Narcissists will use luring tactics not only in the initial phases of getting to know you but will continue to use them with you throughout your relationship.

From the very start, every step they've taken has been part of a well-thought-out process to lure you in, and unfortunately, research indicates that many people who experience online harassment get little support from law enforcement professionals or community organizations, such as their school or university. Lacking support can greatly increase the chances that online harassment will have long-term mental health consequences. You are not crazy if you have experienced cyber-gaslighting. I did, and many others do. Keep a record of what you've experienced and communicate with fellow survivors.

You may feel inclined to avoid the internet after you've experienced harassment. Doing so may reduce distress and help you cope with the experience, but avoiding social media altogether could also make it more difficult to talk to friends and family, which can lead to more isolation.

If you choose to stop using the internet for a time, let your friends and family know what's going on and work out a plan to stay in touch so you don't become isolated. One of the biggest gifts in healing is not being alone, as the emotional support and encouragement of your loved ones can help you get validation for what has happened to you.

THERAPY TIP: PROS AND CONS LIST

Making a list of pros and cons to a certain behavior (e.g., staying in the relationship) can help you gain clarity. This is a tremendous skill for motivating yourself to do what's needed to get free. This requires your logical mind to accomplish. Evaluate what is in it for YOU! This is a subjective exercise designed to help you determine what is best for you. In this case, it will be leave or get wrapped back up into the vortex of this relationship of inevitable harm. Take a piece of paper or use whatever device you like, and create two columns. On the left, at the top, write "reasons to stay"; on the right, at the top, write "reasons to leave." Reference this list as needed if you are having a hard time getting away from the narcissist or maintaining no contact with them.

Chapter 9

"We're Soulmates!"— The Love-Bombing Phase

Cheryl looked out my office window and twisted her ring around her finger. "I don't know, it was like . . . one minute, we are totally in love, then the next minute, everything is my fault. It just doesn't make sense. He'll call me on his way home on a Friday and just say, 'Pack for the weekend' and then he's booked us a luxury resort up the coast—things like that are just, wow. I've never been treated like that! It was like I just had to mention that I liked something and he'd show up with it. But then anytime I didn't thank him enough or whatever, he had some bar that he set that I didn't know; he'd get so mad and tell me I was an ungrateful bitch."

———— <small>⚬∞⚬</small> ————

When it comes to love, there's nothing like the beginning of a new relationship. You and your new boo are totally sweet on each other, you spend all your time together, and things couldn't feel more perfect.

In a healthy relationship, it feels good, but in a relationship with a narcissist, you're likely thinking it's too good to be true, and that's because it is. This phase is the height of fantastical, idealistic showboating during which the narcissist is intense, manipulating their prey with attention and praise. You become indoctrinated in this phase, seduced by the person you have been led to believe is the only one who truly understands you.

Once you agree to be their chosen partner, the narcissist starts demanding and extracting constant adulation and validation from you to satisfy their sense of entitlement and grandiosity. You might even think of it as "love-demanding" rather than love-bombing because it comes at a cost; it is a transaction—and beware. The balance sheet for this transaction is so one-sided that you will never be able to fulfill what the narcissist sees as your debt to them.

WHAT IS LOVE-BOMBING?

The expression "love-bombing" was coined by cult members in the Unification Church of the United States during the 1970s. Psychology professor Margaret Singer reported on the concept in her 1996 book, *Cults in Our Midst*,[1] where she describes love-bombing as a tactic used by cult leaders to feign friendship and interest in new recruits.

In the intervening years, the term has come to refer more generally to any form of such manipulation. "Love-bombing" now most commonly refers to an attempt to influence a person through demonstrations of attention and affection, especially an intense amount of attention and affection during a very short period of time.

The first phase of love-bombing is difficult to differentiate from the honeymoon phase that most relationships experience. The main distinction is that love-bombing is primarily from one partner to the other, a one-sided experience where the narcissist goes overboard with their affection. They do so *until* they have established the semblance of a relationship, but as soon as you cannot give them the constant attention they think they are entitled to, the mask begins to slip. If you have ever said to yourself or others that "When it's good, it's good, but when it's bad, it's bad," you may be dealing with a narcissist.

This is an important distinction to acknowledge because healthy people can do generous and wonderful things for others, but love-bombing is a part of a cycle of abuse. It is used to create a feeling of unity within a group against a society perceived as hostile, such as in a cult, or a feeling of unity with a single person, as in the scenario of a narcissistic intimate partner.

Many of my clients have described the love-bombing phase as one that includes promises of families and homes and a host of other "dreamy" experiences, with the predatory narcissist convincing the victim that their affection is all a sign of "love at first sight." In their unchanging efforts to gain power, pleasure, attention, and profit, narcissists will go to great lengths to attain your trust and help in achieving these goals.

Because our human expectations to repay love-bombing gestures are so high, and because the narcissist regularly rejects any tokens of affection they receive, you may feel that you are not good enough. This shift in your inner dialogue plays right into the trauma bond. Imagine going from the headiest version of yourself—because the narcissist will convince you that the sun rises and sets with you—immediately to a version of yourself that feels lower than garbage. They will build you up tall *just to knock you down*.

The love-bombing phase cannot stand on its own when it comes to narcissistic abuse, though. This is because the narcissist's manipulation and control tactics ramp up when this phase ends and the devaluing phase begins. Psychologist Dale Archer identifies the phases with the acronym IDD: "Intense idealization, Devaluation, Discard (Repeat)."[2]

After the initial excitement and idealization of love-bombing, if you show interest in or care about anything beyond your new partner, the manipulator may show anger or passive-aggressive behavior, or accuse you of selfishness. If you do not comply with their demands, the devaluation stage begins. The abuser withdraws all affection or positive reinforcement and instead punishes you with whatever they feel is appropriate: shouting, berating, mind games, silent treatment, or even physical abuse.

By doing this, the love bomber subtly manipulates you into shutting down your rational mind. Every act of love-bombing is designed to deliver a rush of dopamine into the brain, which habituates you into seeking more dopamine rushes. When these signs of affection are withdrawn, the resulting loss of dopamine hurts even more. As a result, you will begin to feel dependent on your partner, with the expectation that you will continue to receive this form of love.

DIFFERENT TYPES OF LOVE-BOMBING

The basic definition of love-bombing as discussed works in many scenarios, but there are times when love-bombing looks slightly different. In this section, we explore love-bombing from a covert narcissist as well as from a communal narcissist, or cult leader.

Love-Bombing from the Covert Narcissist

As you recall from "Narcissism 101" (page 4), sometimes, narcissists can be covert *and* overt at different times.

The more covert narcissist may use the love-bombing phase to come off as depressed or to portray themselves as the person needing the rescuing. This is a classic example of a narcissist manipulating human emotion for their own gain. Rather than directly building you up during the idealization phase, their game is subtler: taking the fact that people feel good about themselves when they help others and twisting it on its head, they will rely on you to be *their* savior. Then, if you move your focus to something pressing, such as work, health, or even a night out with friends, you become devalued by being blamed when they have a "relapse."

HOW TO KNOW WHETHER YOU'RE BEING LOVE-BOMBED

So, how do you know if your relationship is even real? Is it love-bombing or are they actually that into you? When you're caught in a love-bombing cycle, it can be hard to spot signs of trouble, but the signs are there—if you know where to look.

The key to understanding how love-bombing differs from romantic courtship is to look at what happens after two people are officially a couple. If extravagant displays of affection continue indefinitely, if actions match words and there is no devaluation phase, then it's probably not love-bombing because love-bombing has the motive of hooking you and *then* devaluing you. Love-bombing is only love-bombing when there is ultimate devaluing. It isn't love-bombing if it stands alone.

Do They Respect Your Boundaries?

If you notice that someone bulldozes over your healthy boundaries, have an open conversation with them about how you're feeling and what your boundaries are, and see how they respond. If you voice something that's made you uncomfortable and they take that feedback and incorporate it into changing their behavior moving forward, they probably respect you and care about your relationship. In contrast, if you tell a love bomber you're not okay with their behavior or try to set up healthy boundaries, they likely won't take no for an answer. They may become argumentative, question your line of thinking, or even push you into believing you're wrong for saying no in the first place. If it feels as if a boundary or many boundaries have been crossed, that's a strong sign that your voice isn't being heard and your opinion doesn't matter in the relationship. The love bomber may even be gaslighting you into subscribing to whatever their perspective is.

Because it makes such manipulation tactics as gaslighting easier, narcissists like you better when you're alone. As such, a love-bombing narcissist may buy you gifts and experiences that put you directly into positions where you are alone together. This could mean a spa day with just them, or they may fill up your time with trips and dates to the extent that you are increasingly isolated from friends and family. Sometimes, they could be even more covert and make you feel guilty for doing anything without them; as a result of their getting moody, angsty, or sad, you might purposefully wrap your time up in activities and events that involve them. This will make their imposed isolation feel more subtle, almost as if it were something *you* chose to do.

Do They Demand Your Attention?

Another way to identify a love bomber is if they're in a rush to lock things down. People who love-bomb talk about meeting you as if it has been a lifelong dream.

They may overcommunicate their love for you in day-to-day conversation. A person who love-bombs might check in frequently about what you're doing when they're not around, and pressure you to check in with a similarly high level of frequency. They may do this online by posting too often about their feelings for you in an attempt to gain public acceptance of your relationship. This may be overblown in loving posts on Instagram or Facebook, where they declare their love for you. These efforts actually check a few boxes for them because they are love-bombing you in these moments *and* trying to hurt and devalue their former supplies.

What Sorts of Gifts Do They Give You?

An important key to discerning a true gift from a gift from a narcissist is if it is "needless." A love bomber might shower you with unexpected gifts as tokens of their affection. Although gift-giving is a love language for some people, this becomes a problem when the gifts are unnecessary, unwanted, extravagant, over the top, or make you feel unseen.

Some of the things that the narcissist gifts you may not seem to be things that you might even value or want. The gifts may be things that are highly superficial and not in-line with your desires, such as name-brand bags or shoes when you don't even fancy yourself a bag or shoe kind of person. If you make it known that you don't want these gifts and they keep giving them to you anyway, this is a red flag that you're being love-bombed. These gifts are usually something quite elaborate or expensive, purchased to win you over or lock you down rapidly, and are sometimes based on a narrative that they want the world to see of you or of them.

At other times, they will study you and get you things that fall in-line with what you like and love to further confuse you. While they may occasionally pepper glimpses of authenticity into the relationship, you may feel that they buy you things that serve them, such as by taking you on an extravagant trip where they get to enjoy the "gift" directly.

In the love-bombing phase, you may be given gifts of clothing that may appear gracious and helpful, but this is never the case with a narcissist. They may be grooming you to wear what they think is appropriate, for a variety of different reasons. They may want to control the way that you are viewed by their family or may even want you to dress promiscuously so that you get fired or so that they can objectify you. The way you dress yourself is often a large part of your identity, and they see this as a threat. Sometimes they *do* buy you sentimental things, and this can further confuse you because, on occasion, you will feel seen.

How Do Your Friends and Family Feel?
How Do YOU Feel?

Another litmus test is to check in with your family for a fresh perspective. You'll also want to check in with yourself—and trust that gut feeling you have when something feels wrong.

"Good relationships feel good," states psychologist Alaina Tiani, PhD. "If it feels too good to be true, that's probably an indication that there's something going on. It's important that when those feelings surface, you tune into that instead of pushing it aside."[3]

If you feel overwhelmed, uneasy, or off-balance, this can be an indicator that something is wrong. Sometimes, it's okay to wonder whether you're on the same page as your partner. We all love at different paces and in different stages, and what feels right for someone else may not feel right for you. If you ever communicate these feelings to your partner but they don't reciprocate or respond in healthy, positive ways, these are signs trouble may be brewing.

HOW TO END THE CYCLE OF LOVE-BOMBING

The most effective way to end the cycle of love-bombing is to end the abusive relationship and cut off communication with the narcissist altogether. If this seems too overwhelming, you may need to reduce contact with them slowly and over time. You may need to slowly disallow the narcissist from enticing you with gifts, big promises, or even guilt. Many of my clients practice harm reduction over time, creating distance between them and their abuser. At the end of the love-bombing phase is the start of controlling behavior, but if the love bomber is thwarted or ignored, they either give up their efforts or intensify their love-bombing. The stakes get higher and higher every time you forgive the narcissist, and the punishment becomes harsher and more damaging over time.

In my experience, as well as that of many of my clients, the initial love-bombing phase lasts about four months, but it can carry on for longer. During this time frame, many people express that they felt "something was wrong." According to a survey of five hundred participants conducted by Unfiltered, an organization dedicated to making information about narcissistic abuse widely accessible, the average length of the initial love-bombing phase is between four and eight months.[4] It always circles back around, if given the chance, and it goes on until the person or persons being love-bombed are seduced or get away.

———⊗⊗⊗———

Love-bombing is like a teaser trailer that promises a fluffy romantic story; then, when you buy a ticket, the movie turns out to be a dark survival drama with an ultimately tragic ending.

Oftentimes, the more malignant the narcissist, the shorter the length of the love-bombing phase. This signals the insidious beginning of isolation and control and the deterioration of a survivor's ability to connect with themselves. It happens on repeat, which will be discussed as we move further into the narcissist's playbook of abuse. For now, remember that the two best things you can do in the face of love-bombing are to, first, try to establish healthy boundaries and, second, if those are disrespected, cut off all communication with your narcissistic abuser. If you do not, the cycle will begin again with their love-bombing you back, only to devalue you all over again.

THERAPY TIP:
SETTING HEALTHY BOUNDARIES

As I mentioned earlier, many victims of narcissists don't self-identify as people pleasers but have not set up healthy boundaries at the time their abusers enter their lives. Boundaries are a line that we will not cross in various spaces in our lives; most often, we consciously or unconsciously set physical, emotional, intellectual, material, sexual, and time boundaries.

If you are new to this concept, boundaries may sound restrictive, but they are all really about balance. You can have boundaries and be both open and private; be independent and be dependent; be curious and be suspicious; and be giving and be open to receiving.

When we are developing boundaries, we first need to think about what we want, and then we can discover what we don't want. The following two exercises can help us develop boundaries with others and stay steadfast in that determination.

1. Study and trust.

Knowing what you will accept, and what you will not, begins with studying yourself and trusting yourself. Have a clear understanding of what you want from an interaction or a relationship and communicate this clearly as needed. To get started, make a list of things that you want in friends, partners, and your career as a way to remind yourself of some of the values you are looking for. Review this list regularly.

2. Practice holding your line.

The next time you find yourself in an uncomfortable situation, recall your list of values. Give yourself permission to say no, clearly and strongly. Do not apologize for saying no, and do not be vague. Similarly, the next time someone crosses a line that makes you feel uncomfortable and does not resonate with your values list, let them know that it will not be something you will continue to endure, or you will put space between you and that person. Try saying something like "That doesn't work for me."

Above all, stay true to yourself.

Chapter 10

"Jekyll & Hyde"— The Mask-Slipping Phase

My client Jane tells me that she married her ex-husband at a castle in England. On her wedding night, her then-husband attempted to strangle her. She claims that she had always felt something was off about him, but when she saw this other side of him, she was rocked to her core. "How can this be the person claiming to love me so much? Who is this person?"

———— ✖ ————

After you have been love-bombed, the narcissist will begin to show you parts of their true selves.

Welcome to the mask-slipping phase. Narcissists often go to great lengths to maintain their false persona in public, but when the mask slips, revealing the ruinous Mr. Hyde to their "good guy" Dr. Jekyll personality, it is often only a matter of time before they will seek to discard and destroy you. You will see their true selves during this phase, and it will be a shocking contrast to their previous performance as the love bomber.

The mask-slipping phase is where the narcissist becomes more brazen, less insidious. This is the phase where they realize they have "gotten" you, and it could be because they became engaged to you, married you, moved you in, hired you, got you pregnant, or have some other hierarchical role whereby they are in control of your life. They have devalued you enough, made you vulnerable enough, and have enough control over you to actually show you who they are. The fact that they are tiring of the facade tells you that they may be nearing the discard phase, and ultimately the postseparation abuse that follows. Keep in mind, though, that a lot of them can keep up the charade for many years, appearing to be a loving person to the public while being a miserable soul behind closed doors.

The narcissist in your life may build themselves up by breaking you down and one-upping you in front of others in a way that feels very shameful and embarrassing. They may flirt with someone else in front of you in their efforts to turn on the charm; they may even compare you to others to make you feel "less than."

All along the way, they will gaslight and manipulate you; they may beam with adoration for you in one breath, then replace it with a scowl within a fraction of a second. The speed of this transformation is disconcerting, and all efforts to get them back to the other version of themselves will fail, even as you blame yourself for it all. Disorienting you and keeping you off-balance maintains your compliance with their bad behavior because, if you are constantly second-guessing yourself, they are more likely to (a) get away with whatever they want, and (b) reinforce your reliance on them for "reality checking." They build you up to break you down, over and over and over again.

They have to show you this side of themselves to see how much you will tolerate. Over time, they will turn up the dial and increase your exposure to their dark side. Eventually, the narcissistic manipulator will have no further need for pretense and will toy with you, in the mask-slipping phase, just for sport. They will try to turn everyone against you to make themselves look like the victim. They will use your friends, family, and even strangers to push their agenda. They will go from the perfect partner to a chronic liar and circular converser. They use language, not to communicate, but to obscure the truth and to play mind games. During this phase, the narcissist will be moody and antagonistic. They will engage in ultimatums, walkouts, blowups, threats, accusations, and the silent treatment. You may not be able to find them for prolonged clips of time and will wonder what you did wrong. But remember, the narcissist is often anxious or on edge specifically because they are afraid they will get caught in their lies. In the mask-slipping phase, the narcissist will often use projection to accuse others of the behaviors they are actually engaging in. You may discover they have a hidden life full of affairs, sexual deviancy, drug abuse, and illegalities. As we've covered, the narcissist is terrified of being alone, so they often juggle multiple victims and multiple sources of attention. As such, they may be in the love-bombing phase with someone else or keep an ex or mistress on the back burner, an ugly truth you may learn about during this phase. Ultimately, the real person will emerge and eclipse the mask.

IS MASK-SLIPPING A CHOICE?

Not all people with narcissistic personality disorder (NPD) are necessarily Machiavellian enough to play mask-slipping as a planned game. The vast majority simply tire of their fake personas and begin to see little value in playing the role anymore. When they are having a good day, they can wear the mask with ease, but when they feel insecure, the mask will slip, and they will act grandiose, dismissive of and abusive toward other people. If triggered, they will overreact, devalue, scream at, and blame their victim for anything and everything. They are known to threaten to destroy the lives of their victims during the mask-slipping phase. After they explode and become abusive, it is usually pointless to confront them about their bad behavior. If you confront them, they will attack you.

HOW IS MASK-SLIPPING DIFFERENT
FROM GETTING COMFY?

We all do a lot to make a strong first impression; we work to put our best foot forward when we meet someone new. But mask-slipping is not just having a bad day or letting a new love interest see us without makeup or allowing ourselves to slowly be revealed, warts and all; those are all natural occurrences as healthy relationships progress.

We can all be vulnerable, moody, and shift between feeling good and feeling down or irritable, based on a number of variables, including hormones, hunger, exhaustion, fear, and frustration, but mask-slipping is different. This is a pathological perversion of the way most neurotypical people relax as they get to know you better. This is someone turning on a different version of themselves to play a role in different scenarios.

With mask-slipping, you see whispers of the real person who has been manipulating you. In other words, we all may become lax and change a bit after the honeymoon phase of a relationship, but this is more about the narcissist dropping whatever chameleon-like version of themselves that they had crafted *just for you*! This fake persona was always a con job, and the narcissist will ultimately not want to play that role any longer.

Here are some common examples of the masks that can slip.

Lovesick Romeo (a.k.a. the love bomber). The narcissist is extremely convincing when they are playing this role and may even fool themselves.

Dedicated Parent. Despite all the abuse that the narcissist puts their family through, they will portray themselves as an amazing parent in public. Whether "mother of the year," with pictures of the "perfect family" displayed prominently on social media; or the soccer dad, always the life of the party; or the church-going and devoted worshipper in the family, they can be the biggest bully behind closed doors, creating toxicity and chaos behind the scenes.

The Victim. A covert or vulnerable narcissist presents as shy, wounded, humble, and insecure, but underneath that disguise is a self-centered, entitled, yet miserable soul. They slowly construct an image in the minds of others that they are not just a good person but a noble martyr, lying about what they believe and what they have done. When they are misunderstood or something doesn't go their way, they will play the victim and portray others as the abusers, even calling them narcissists.

Charismatic Leader. Narcissists often finds themselves in leadership roles, which they enjoy because it feeds their motivational goals of status, power, and attention. To achieve and maintain these roles, they develop the skill of being charming early on. This is transactional; charisma with a purpose—they turn it on and off according to what they think needs to be witnessed by a certain person. They shine brightest when others are watching because they only need this tool with an audience.

There is always an agenda, but it is hard to detect because they have been practicing it for so long. When you meet a Charismatic Leader, you will likely think they are popular, nice, intriguing, smart, and loyal. You may even have been a little starstruck or have wondered why someone with their high accolades has taken such a strong interest in you. This is because they are masters of first impressions. They are often well groomed, covered in cologne, sexualized, inquisitive, touchy-feely, good at making eye contact, complimentary, warm, friendly, seemingly intuitive, ready to share "coincidences" with you—to put it bluntly: they are overall good actors.

Generous Philanthropist. Some narcissists are ostentatiously generous and can be found donating turkeys around Thanksgiving. They give of their time and money because it enhances their sense of grandiosity and allows them to exert control over the beneficiaries. They now feel as if they own, even if it is in a small way, the people involved in the organization they have donated to, even parts of the organization itself. By allocating funds or other gifts to charities, the narcissist now knows where they stand and can rest easy that they can do what they like without anyone from said organization pushing back against any bad behaviors. Additionally, it could anger past victims, who know the narcissist does not care about a certain charity, to learn that they are forcing people to celebrate them at functions and galas in spite of the disdain the narcissist holds for this particular cause, and this works for the narcissist because they are so vindictive.

Devoted Spouse. The narcissist pretends to be a stellar spouse and will often play the victim of the *actual* victim by calling their husband or wife crazy. As with the Dedicated Parent, most other people don't know what happens behind closed doors.

Spiritual Guru. Whether at the center of a cult or in a cult of one, many narcissists pretend to be spiritual gurus or people who possess some special enlightened thinking. Like many gurus, they demand complete obedience from their flock. That flock, in the case of the narcissist in a family dynamic, is composed of their spouse, children, friends, colleagues, and other acquaintances.

The less accomplished they are in reality, the more spiritual bullshit the Spiritual Guru narcissist will peddle. The members of the narcissist's mini-cult have to deal with their imposing on their flock a shared psychosis with persecutory delusions, fake enemies, mythical narratives, conspiracy theories, superstitions, apocalyptic scenarios, and psychic beliefs. This is all to get their victims as far away from reality and scientific data as possible. The "guru's" control is based on ambiguity, unpredictability, fuzziness, and ever-shifting whims designed to alter their followers' sensibilities about what is right and wrong. The narcissistic guru claims to be infallible, superior, talented, skillful, omnipotent, and omniscient.

High-Academic Intellectual. The "cerebral" narcissist, or self-proclaimed "intellectual" narcissist, will often monopolize conversations to focus on their intellectual achievements. Sometimes they embellish their accolades to make themselves look even better than they are. They roll their eyes when others are speaking; cut people off or talk over them; and even make such comments as "You don't know what you're talking about" or "I know better."

They may insult people who they believe are inferior to them and use language that is degrading and critical. While it may seem counterintuitive, cerebral narcissists will often put themselves in the company of other highly intelligent people. This way, they can boast to others about being included in these environments. The only real thing they are smart about is they are socially perceptive, which makes it easy for them to read others and use that information to exploit.

Friendly Neighbor. The narcissist next door may portray themselves as a pillar of the community, even as you notice certain things happening behind closed doors or overhear them arguing with their children or spouse. They often seek the opportunity to start a conversation with you, but it never feels as if they're actually interested in anything you have to say. Conversations with them instead turn into a monologue about how brilliant or successful they are. They may use heavy surveillance at their home, or come and go at odd hours. They also seem to have a problem with boundary crossing. They're always coming over uninvited or asking personal questions that make you feel uncomfortable. They are also usually the only ones on the street who do not follow the rules, such as parking illegally, refusing to pick up garbage or clean up after their pets, or blaring music late into the night.

NARCISSISTIC COLLAPSE

The mask-slipping phase typically happens because a narcissist doesn't want to uphold their fake exterior any longer. Meanwhile, **narcissistic collapse** occurs when a narcissist's ability to uphold their grandiose, confident image, or mask, while they still feel a need to wear it, is threatened. As a result, they can become enraged, impulsively and intensely lashing out or in some other way causing harm to others.

Some narcissists will collapse as they age because they feel they no longer possess their beautiful exterior or athletic abilities. Some will collapse after losing money in the stock market or in other business failings. Some may collapse after they are discovered to be cheating on their spouse by their spouse or by their children. Some may fall ill from all the chaos that they have brought into their lives and have a heart attack or stroke from the resulting stress.

Whatever the reason, when their bubble of omnipotence bursts, they feel as if the ground beneath them has disappeared, which can be incredibly destabilizing. Without their grandiose bullshit to use as a crutch, they may sink into a shame-based depression in which they are afraid of the future and can no longer function in the present.

Some may dial up their abuse of their spouse or children during and after their collapse. Some may even become homicidal or suicidal. Many turn to drugs or alcohol to abuse them to cope with their feelings of incompetency. They may seek therapy at this time, due to severe anxiety and/or depressive symptoms and an inability to function at work or at home. Many check into a rehab facility to "work" on themselves, but this is just a front to play the victim or to become a martyr. If you remain a supply in the narcissist's life during a mask slip or narcissistic collapse, the kicker is that the narcissist will make you believe that it's *all your fault*.

———— ⚬⚭⚬ ————

In the end, whether due to collapse or their own weariness with playing a role, wearing a mask is not sustainable for the narcissist. The stress that they put themselves under, due to playing a role every day, becomes an impossible thing to keep up, so they begin to burn out, which likely will lead to the discard phase.

Life lived behind a mask means that the narcissist will feel increasingly boxed in or on the verge of exposure or collapse, and because of this, the narcissist may move—across jobs, regions, careers, families, relationships, and other interests—with a frightening fluidity. They are always on the run from the truth of what they are. Keeping up appearances is next to impossible, so as soon as they think the jig is up or feel that a particular supply no longer serves them, they are *out*. When this happens, the narcissist won't care *at all*. They lack sentimentality and see nothing and no one other than their own needs and how to meet them, so there is no way they are going to become attached to Little Suzy's first piece of artwork in kindergarten. (I suppose if Little Suzy's artwork were some prodigious chance to get her into a special school, then maybe the narcissist would care—but only if the school's principal was someone they wanted to golf with.) Unless it serves them, they don't care. The mask-slipping and the discard phases of the narcissistic cycle of abuse can be particularly difficult for survivors to cope with, both in those horrible moments and after. It is my hope that this chapter and the next one will help you be forewarned and forearmed, and that they will give you the tools you need to move forward and to successfully discard your own dead weight—the narcissistic abuser who has been holding you back.

THERAPY TIP: DIVERSIFY

Isolation is never good for you, especially not when you start to see the narcissist's mask slipping. This may mean that the narcissist is getting ready to discard you, and you will need to lean on others to get through that.

Increase your support system and share the truth. When you reach out to our support system to share with them our reality—what is happening; what you know; and what you've seen, witnessed, and experienced—you are further integrating the truth into your mind. This can be the antidote to the gaslighting and cognitive dissonance you are experiencing.

It can be difficult to gather the courage to do this, but it is important to do so. The more you stay quiet and downplay your realities, the more likely it is that the seeds of doubt will grow in your mind. The narcissist has spent a lot of energy combatting your connection to friends and family, for precisely this purpose. You may avoid telling friends and family what you are enduring because you are afraid that they won't want to hear it anymore, but you need external validation from your support system to build your internal confidence, especially when you are the victim of gaslighting. You can reduce the psychological and emotional hold that a gaslighter has on you when you share your truths with safe people.

If your friends and family are tired of hearing about it, *find others who will listen*. Trusted professionals, mental health hotlines, and confidential support groups can be good places to start. It is so important to continue to express what you are experiencing, so that you do not internalize the garbage that the narcissist is trying to put into your mind. That way, when you begin to see the mask slipping, you will not lose your support system—the very thing that will help save you in the end.

You'll find suggestions for getting help in the Resources section, pages 275–277.

Chapter 11

"Kicked to the Curb"— The Discard Phase

My client Paulina started seeing me after her ex abandoned her, her son, and their two cats. She told me, "I didn't actually know what was happening. He wasn't returning my calls or texts; one day I saw him with another woman—and clearly they were involved. I didn't know what was happening to us. My son cried for days; he wore my ex's shirt—wouldn't take it off because he missed him so much. I mean, how do I tell my kid that this guy, who he felt was like a father, is . . ." She trailed off. The description she gave me of how he took the new supply on holidays and to concerts, while ignoring her cries for help, was heart-wrenching. "Vanessa, he put our belongings on the street."

F irst, they put you on a pedestal. Then, they pick at you, engaging in passive-aggressive punishing tactics, such as the silent treatment. Finally, they discard you like garbage.

What went wrong?

The vicissitude of the discard phase can happen many times over the course of a narcissistic relationship, so let me open this chapter by emphasizing that there are two versions of the discard: the one where you get "benched" until the narcissist comes back around to you, and the "final discard." Both versions can make you feel as if you have been thrown out like trash, but it is important to understand that the discard is not always as permanent as it sounds; that is, it is not always the final blow. This is, more often than not, a "temporary discard"—just a part of the cycle of abuse until they really do discard, or leave, you forever.

WHY THE NARCISSIST DISCARDS THEIR SUPPLY

The discard phase is where the narcissist either disappears or orchestrates their own abandonment. Sometimes, this seems to be prompted by the victim asking for something like compromise, reciprocity, empathy, integrity, honesty, or healthier boundaries, but remember, neither the discard nor any other aspect of narcissistic abuse is your fault.

Here are some of the real reasons that the narcissist may discard you:

- You were too difficult for them to control.
- You were easily manipulated by them, causing them to look down upon you.
- You no longer fuel their ego, so they've moved on to someone else.
- You figured them out.
- You may not be able to help them any further with their life goals.
- They feel that they can "level up" and move on to someone "better."
- They want to focus on something they deem more interesting.
- They want to see you beg for them back.
- They want to punish you.
- You lost your "luster" and are no longer the "perfect" partner.
- You no longer play along with their fantasy.

The discard and its resulting blowout argument come with a sense of blindsidedness that leaves the victim feeling ashamed, guilty, and filled with grief. You might also feel a sense of dread; oftentimes, this is your gut telling you that the narcissist has already moved on to their next target while you grieve alone, isolated from friends and family.

The disorienting part of a temporary discard is that you will struggle to understand why the narcissist keeps coming back for more, not to mention why your fights happen on repeat. Narcissists love a fight, plain and simple. They will bait you, poke you, and incite you to shout and fight back. They will drop politically polarizing comments and insults into conversations or create conflict between you and others to get that much-needed attention. They will dredge up any old argument, just to get you exasperated. They feed off your energy, and so, in this phase, they may "discard" you just to have you beg them to forgive you, all the while knowing they are doing it just to get a rise out of you.

Narcissists frequently come back to existing sources of supply after a temporary discard in a move called "hoovering." They need someone on hand to give them a steady supply of attention, so they will suck you back (like a vacuum) into their web from time to time. They like the idea that, even after time apart, they can still control your emotions and energy.

When you don't take the bait, it is actually frustrating for them. This is a big reason that I coach my clients to not be reactive at any time. If you don't react, the narcissist may reveal themselves, becoming increasingly agitated. When they do, you can begin to chronicle their bad behavior to protect and insulate yourself from their future harm, up to and including court battles and other forms of legal abuse. Put simply, you mustn't feed the monster.

THE TRAUMA OF THE DISCARD

You may not realize that you were being traumatized long before the discard because the extreme highs of the love-bombing phase and the extreme lows of the devaluing phase will likely lead to a trauma bond, but the final discard is where you may really begin to awaken to the trauma. After a discard, you may spend a good deal of time hoping they will come back around. The reality of that not happening can be extremely traumatic and could lead you to a very dark place.

The discard is not likely the only trauma you have experienced but a culmination of all you have endured. The following criteria apply to adults, adolescents, and children older than six years when diagnosing post-traumatic stress disorder (PTSD). If you have experienced them, you have likely been traumatized by your narcissistic abuser's actions, including during the discard phase.

- Exposure to actual or threatened death, serious injury, or sexual violence, whether this exposure is experienced directly by you or you witness it happening to others
- Experiencing repeated or extreme exposure to aversive details of the traumatic event(s), such as first responders' collecting human remains or police officers repeatedly exposed to details of child abuse
- Recurrent, involuntary, and intrusive distressing memories of the traumatic events
- Nightmares, night terrors, and difficulty sleeping
- Intense or prolonged psychological distress at exposure to internal or external cues that symbolize or resemble an aspect of the traumatic event(s) we experienced; an example of this may be when a rape victim has intimacy issues with a new partner
- Persistent avoidance of stimuli associated with the traumatic event(s), beginning after the traumatic event(s) occurred; this might look like avoiding geographic locations where you may run into an abuser
- Inability to remember an important aspect of the traumatic event(s) or an inability to focus or concentrate; many victims of narcissistic abuse will dissociate from their memories as a way to avoid the pain that comes from thinking about them
- Irritability

- Hypervigilance or an exaggerated startle response; my son and I always joke about how if you turn the corner in my house and I don't anticipate it, I will jump directly out of my socks with fear

Narcissistic abuse can also lead to complex post-traumatic stress disorder (C-PTSD), which has all the symptoms of PTSD, plus additional symptoms, such as:

- Difficulty regulating emotions, which can manifest into extreme anger, depression, suicidal thoughts, and quick, extreme mood swings
- Dissociation, or feeling detached from oneself
- Intense feelings of shame and guilt
- Distorted perceptions of the abuser, such as ascribing all the power to this person, being obsessed with the abuser, or becoming preoccupied with revenge
- Some studies have found that victims of this kind of trauma experience what is termed a *mental death*, meaning they have lost their pretrauma sense of identity; a "dark night of the soul"

Beyond the trauma, it is also important to understand why victims have a hard time liberating themselves from these relationships. There are physiological and neurobiological reasons victims cannot let their narcissistic abusers go. The brain is altered by trauma and repeated abuse cycles; the victim becomes addicted to the dopamine hits that happen whenever the narcissist pulls them closer and gives them just enough relief to keep them hooked.[1] This is cult programming, brainwashing, with a dose of capture-bonding tossed in for extra staying power.[2]

When the narcissist pushes you away, even if temporarily, you suffer, hoping to get release from their purgatory of isolation and rejection. You become a junkie, with the fear of loss and the need for approval keeping you bound to your abuser.[3] If you do not lose everything by your own decision to choose the narcissist over everyone and everything else, then they will cause rifts in all your relationships, so that you belong to them completely. They become the center of your universe, and you, in turn, rationalize why you had to push people out of your life.

In the end, you will inevitably lose the narcissist and the life they promised; you will have fallen for their future-faking, which kept you hopeful, kept you thinking that your dreams can come true if you hold on just a little longer. So, all your eggs go into the narcissist's basket, and sooner or later, they will run away with your eggs *and* your basket to start the cycle again.

An abusive relationship is traumatic when you're in it, but the trauma that comes after the abusive relationship has ended is realized because you have lost the one person who has come to define your worth. On top of these already serious threats to your mental health, you may be financially or professionally dependent on your abuser, so you may also experience financial losses or professional setbacks. While the discard brings the inherent trauma of the relationship to the surface, remember that, in the long run, you will be better off without your abuser.

THE FINAL DISCARD

It is hard for so many long-term victims of narcissistic abuse to comprehend that after a year, five years, fifteen years, or even thirty, your abuser may kick you to the curb—and in the most ruthless way imaginable. Because the discard has been a temporary part of an ongoing cycle for so long, you will not know the relationship is truly over until the final discard has already happened. (Oftentimes, you realize it because you find yourself in a courtroom battle with your ex.) The final discard can feel like you've had the rug ripped out from under you. You may be left without a job, home, money, or friends and family because the narcissist has worked toward destroying you throughout the entire relationship, right under your nose and without your even knowing it.

The narcissist believes their own fantasy version of the relationship in the beginning, and before long, their partner has joined them to believe it too. It is intense and colorful and larger than life because it is a concept not built in actuality. It is very hard to go up against the magical and delusional plans that a master manipulator peddles to you and seemingly for you. Once you awaken from the glittery fever dream that was the narcissist's world, you have to learn how to live in the harsh glare of the real world, far removed from the love bubble they caged you in.

The loss of this shared fantasy is no easy thing to traverse. You will doubt everything around you, and even distrust yourself for a long time. One of the main reasons that the final discard can annihilate the victim is that it triggers old childhood wounds, a combination of present pain and past, unresolved pain. It is a reminder of the hurt you felt when someone rejected you, abandoned you, or neglected you during your early developmental years. It is an all-too-familiar feeling of invalidation and invisibility swaddled in shame and disbelief. The ensnarement and subsequent mutual psychosis that the victim experienced during the luring and love-bombing phases, as well as the loss of that poisonous bond, can cause an existential crisis that many cannot come back from. The predatory narcissist has hypnotized them, sedated them, and tricked them into a state of helplessness.

Not only will the narcissist use the final discard to burn all your resources, but also all the bridges you built together. This is one of the reasons that victims of the narcissistic discard suffer from PTSD—they have become addicted to the highs that come from the "altitudes" of the hyperdoting phase and wrecked by the blow of the rejection of the final discard.

The most unlucky victims are the ones that are hijacked, devoured, and "symbiotically" absorbed into the narcissistic relationship, only to be expelled as a fraction of the person they used to be with little understanding of what happened and no idea how to fix it.

Although some victims of narcissistic abuse do not ever fully recover, many others do. They find a new lease on life and can find the god winks or silver linings after the discard, but this is no small task or quick remedy. In later chapters, we will go into more about healing. For now, try to think of this rebirth as similar to that of people who have a near-death experience in which they clinically die for a minute or two before coming back to life. These people often express that they have been changed by their experience. They have seen the other side, and so they can never be who they were before. They have passed through the valley of the shadow of death, and they have a chance to turn their pain into power.

After it becomes apparent that the latest discard was the *last* one, the only thing to do is get up and start the arduous task of inventing a new identity, a new and improved 2.0 version of you. You owe it to yourself. Do not be afraid. Life can be so much better than it was before or during your relationship with the narcissist. They have made you think that they were the one in charge, but what do we know about them? *They are liars.* Nothing can ever harm you as much as what you have just survived. The next part of your life can be whatever you want it to be.

WHEN YOU LEAVE THE NARCISSIST

Although a victim of abuse voluntarily choosing to discard their narcissist is not as common as when the narcissist discards their supplies, it does happen. It did with me. I left my abuser. I only beat him to it, but I did. If you are reading this in the midst of a relationship, know that you can do it. It is not easy, but you can do it. If you are reading this after the fact, I'm proud of you and hope these next chapters will continue to support you.

People may tire of the roller-coaster ride or find out about their partner's double life—infidelities, lies, drug abuse, gambling, and more—and want to get away from the relationship. They may gain a bit of clarity during a bout of narcissist-imposed silent treatment or a discard-related break. When this happens, you might hold your nose, jump in the water, and flee.

Choosing to leave your narcissistic abuser can be extremely scary, and this is often when a survivor of abuse is in the most danger. This is because, while the narcissist cares about optics and attention, they care the most about *winning.* This "loss" (your leaving them before they discard you) will put you on the receiving end of some seriously scary revenge tactics.

The narcissist who gets left is retaliation in human form. Narcissists (along with sociopaths and psychopaths) believe that the world owes them something, and this "dueness" will lead to massive rage if they do not get what they feel they deserve. The narcissist feels justified in raging back, using legal abuse, stalking, slander, or exploitation of private information that they have harbored in the imminent smear campaign.

A narcissist's vengeful nature often translates into postseparation abuse. The narcissist is like the spinning spotlight at a prison yard. If you are trying to escape, and you duck, the light (guard/narcissist) in the tower may catch someone else that is trying to dodge their punishments. You are not alone in the prison yard. They are always punishing someone. When a narcissist feels wronged, all their own painful thoughts, feelings, and emotions get triggered and compromise their emotional stability. Once this happens, they will use projection as a defense mechanism, blaming everyone else for their inability to look inward: *I am not the unlovable, unwanted, inadequate, worthless, and weak one; they are*. This blame will translate into their pointing the finger at you and, depending on the resources they have, this could be deadly. They may try to bait you so that you become reactive, and then they will record your reactions, or they could intimidate you by breaking a restraining order.

Sometimes, they do this *just* to get you to spend money on attorneys' fees, which brings us to one of the narcissist's favorite retaliatory tactics: legal abuse. In many cases, they will even the score by forcing you into lengthy court battles so they can continue to exert control and rob you of your time, money, and energy. In a custody battle, they may portray themselves as the good parent, all in an attempt to harm you in the most vicious of ways: by taking your children from you and turn them against you. This is the worst part I have ever seen in all of my work with my clients: the grooming and ruination of their children as well as the domestic terrorism of the family court judicial system. We will get into this more later.

Yes, leaving your narcissist can be extremely scary, and rebuilding your life after they've discarded you can feel like you've hit rock bottom. But here's a secret the narcissist doesn't want you to know: it gets better.

In the end, you are the life source and magic that they desire, and you always were. This is what freedom feels like: a gift. Your discard may not feel like the bequest that it is at the time, but it will. You will begin to see the first-rate gratification of overcoming the seemingly insurmountable pain and agony that comes from having your soul blasted away. You will gain a newfound trust in yourself and your abilities.

Not that it will be easy—*it will not.* It will tear you to shreds, but then, in the aftermath, you will become the person you were always meant to be. You will become the soldier and sure-footed savior you always needed others to be for you. You will rise, and you will become the best version of yourself.

THERAPY TIP: COPE WITH DISCARD

Most of the trauma of a narcissistic relationship, for so many victims, comes after the discard. To deal with this experience, many victims report needing to get back in touch with who they were before they met their abuser. Try the following tips as you start this challenging journey for yourself.

- **Try to remember who you were before this relationship.** This can also help you break the trauma bond, which we will talk more about in a future chapter. When I left my abusive relationship, I had really and truly forgotten who I was. I was no longer the funny and goofy girl I had always prided myself on being, but I was determined to find her again. Similarly, my beloved son had lost himself in the relationship. While he wasn't as traumatized as I was after the relationship because he was away at college, he was hurt by the gaslighting, lies, and confusion that he had endured. He and I sat down, and I described to him how I was feeling and how he needed to find the guy he was before this all happened. The reminder of who Anthony was *before* this relationship became a "ground zero" for him to find his footing and step back into the reality of his own identity, not the fantasy of what my abuser wanted him to be.

- **Learn or relearn how healthy relationships develop and exist,** which is often more slowly and with less fire and drama than narcissistic relationships. Look to surround yourself with friends or potential partners that exhibit the following characteristics: empathy, honesty, trust, respect, open communication with compromise, and no imbalance of power.

- **Surround yourself with genuinely supportive people.** Relationships with people who have narcissistic tendencies can leave you feeling isolated and questioning your reality. Spending time with people who genuinely care about your well-being can help you reincorporate healthier perspectives into your life and regain your sense of equilibrium. So much healing can come from being around people who validate you and celebrate your victories.

- **Reflect on the factors that attracted you to a relationship with this person in the first place.** You may be surprised to find that the narcissist resembled a figure in your childhood, such as a parent who was unavailable to you. Much of the healing comes in this space, which we will talk about much more in a future chapter.

Chapter 12

Planted Seeds Grow into Trees—The Smear Campaign Phase

It's my third session with Jodi, and she tells me about how she believed her new boyfriend had pinched her dog. She noticed that the dog yelped when he was petting her and that the dog had never done that before. When she confronted her boyfriend, he would go to her friends and express concern for Jodi's well-being, stating that he was a bit concerned about her. When Jodi tried to take her friends aside and explain, they thought she seemed hysterical and unstable because it sounded crazy—why would anyone, especially a new boyfriend, harm her dog JUST to make her look crazy? Ultimately, Jodi was a victim of her boyfriend's planting seeds that turned into trees in the smear campaign.

A smear campaign occurs when the narcissist systematically villain-izes you through lies and deception, so they can gain the support of potential accomplices and destroy your reputation in the process. The campaign is used to discredit another person by hijacking the narrative of a relationship. It is a manipulative tactic they use to insulate themselves from the truth that may potentially come out—the truth that they are the problem. One of the most painful characteristics of the smear campaign is that, once it is over, the narcissist is left with an army of accomplices, many of whom were originally your closest friends. You lose your support system while the narcissist has acquired accomplices to further trauma-tize you. All of this can result in a severe disadvantage for you in family court systems, child custody evaluations, and other legal matters. With more people and resources on their side, the narcissist gains more power to exploit and terrorize you. The narcissist needs their smear campaign or they would lose their power.

This tactic works, for the most part, because narcissists are highly convincing salespeople. Through a combination of projecting blame, play-ing savior, and playing victim, they can goad your existing support sys-tem to alienate and shame you in a way you would have previously found unfathomable. The narcissist uses their accomplices to push you into the corner and, unfortunately, in many cases, to the brink of suicide. Many of my clients tell me that their abuser expressed having the ultimate goal of driving them to suicide. This feels like ultimate control to the narcissist, and they may even tell their victims that they will get them to the point that they will want to kill themselves.

The level of manipulation behind a smear campaign is extraordinary. To prove one is happening, you need to take an irrefutable, impartial, and evidence-based approach to gathering data on your abuser.

Narcissists view a breakup as a war that they are determined to win. They will play the role of the victim while actively besmirching you. They will use the judicial system to press false charges and file lawsuits, to bully

and intimidate you. They will threaten your career, reputation, and relationships through fear, intimidation, threats, stalking, malicious prose-
cution, legal abuse, and tortuous interference, as well as exploitation and
manipulation of children and finances. They will try to take custody of
shared children, not because they care but to harm you.

In the narcissistic cycle of abuse, the smear campaign phase is the
most dangerous to you because you are under attack when you are at
your most vulnerable. In other words, you are dealing with a nervous system that has been so compromised that you may not have the strength to
endure any more than you are already dealing with. It is almost impossible
for you to process what has happened to you, and yet you are expected, not
only to put one foot in front of the other day in and day out, but to fight
for everything you have (including in many instances, your children in a
courtroom). Because your friends and family haven't lived with the narcissist, it's nearly impossible for them to see through the narcissist's lies and
truly validate your experience. As a result, some people have to cut and
run, to save themselves from their abuser—sometimes even leaving their
precious children behind.

If you suspect your partner is perpetrating such a campaign against
you, it may be helpful to know that a narcissistic smear campaign is:

- **Disproportionate.** Smear campaigns are much more than the
  occasional talking behind someone's back. These are persistent,
  consistent, and excessive acts to harm another person's reputation,
  such as going after their career, as well as the career and reputation
  of their family and friends, or trying to damage relationships with
  friends, family, or colleagues at work.
- **Vengeful.** The narcissist may seek revenge because they believe
  they have been grievously injured in some way.
- **Purposeful.** Their actions are not made by mistake, despite what
  they might say to others about "just being concerned." They are
  engaging in this smear campaign to destroy you, which they think
  will make them look better.

- **Persistent.** Even when faced with backlash, the narcissist's behavior persists. Narcissists do not let up. In fact, they will dig their heels in deeper if they think that they are losing control of the smear campaign.
- **Projected.** Many narcissists project their worst qualities onto others. If they lie and steal, they accuse their target of doing those things.

THE SEEDS OF THE SMEAR CAMPAIGN

The narcissist starts laying the groundwork for the smear campaign long before they discard you. During the relationship, when they realize that they are no longer interested in your supply, they will start by dropping hints to family and friends via innuendo and inference. Early on, usually by the time the devaluing stage starts, they plant seeds by telling people that things between you are not going as well as they had hoped. They might say that you "have changed" or are "drinking too much" or seem "mentally unstable." They may tell your family that you are not a good cook or lie to friends by saying they think you are sleeping around. You might see them push your buttons in front of others to get you to react. They do this so that, when they finally discard and smear you, their lies will be believed. They may start doing this early on by asking the children, friends, or other family members, such things as "Do you think Mom is doing drugs?" or "Do you think Mom is acting normal?" and so the seeds of doubt are planted.

The forethought that goes into the smear campaign cannot be understated because it is extremely hard to believe and yet it is absolutely true. The narcissist may even tell you that family members have noticed things about you and have voiced concerns. They do this to confuse you and make you think something is wrong with you (a key part of the devaluation process). Meanwhile, the truth is that they have spread lies to your family members and friends behind your back. If you push back against this, they will become defensive.

THE SMEAR CAMPAIGN AFTER
THE DISCARD

The foundation for the smear campaign is laid from the early days of the narcissistic relationship. Then, at the final discard, the entire house of lies is erected. At this point, the narcissist will go full bore, sharing unflattering bits of information they have tucked away or crafting full-blown lies to use against you.

When the relationship ends, especially if you ended it, they will begin to seek revenge against you. To villainize you, the narcissist will use lies, exaggerations, and embellishments of the truth to instill doubt about your reputation among others. Sometimes, they will even tell you what they are doing. They may say things like:

- "I am going to make it so any judge will deny you access to the kids."
- "I will get you kicked off the board."
- "You will never be able to step foot into the children's elementary school after I am done with you."
- "Nobody is going to believe you."
- "I will destroy you."
- And, perhaps most chillingly, "I will make it so you will want to kill yourself."

WHY NARCISSISTS USE SMEAR CAMPAIGNS

Their reasons usually revolve around a need for revenge, a goal to discredit you, a fear of being exposed, and their own lack of compassion and empathy. They always have to get ahead of and one-up their adversaries, so they are very forward thinking; they try to stay in a position of controlling the way people think about most things, especially them.

WHEN YOU START TO DATE AGAIN

It is important to be prepared for the narcissist's reaction before you start dating someone else because it can quickly become treacherous. Being prepared can help you protect yourself from this misery. When you do feel safe enough to date again, be aware that the narcissist will likely initiate a new wave of smear tactics. They will chase away and intimidate your new partners because the idea of your having the ability to move on and find happiness is the supreme trigger for them, and they will work tirelessly to sabotage its potential for you. They may reach out to your new love interest, even if it is many years after your breakup, to try to create problems between you two.

They may feel jealous and threatened, and may send out passive-aggressive texts or calls to your new companion to try to defile your name. Make it clear to your new honey that things are over between you and your ex, and that there is no chance of your getting back together. Keep in mind that you may have to share parts of your story to further highlight what you have endured, even providing education around how narcissistic abusers operate.

———⊗⊗⊗———

Narcissistic smear campaigns are a bloody, gruesome battle, but when the smoke clears, the god wink in the aftermath is that you will discover something poetic and beautiful: true friends.

Some people in your circle may say things to you like "Why did you stay?" or "I don't get it. He never did anything bad to me." These are people who do not understand narcissistic abuse, and you will have to decide if it is worth your energy to explain what it is to them. I personally try to explain what this is to people because I do not feel that things will change without education, but even these efforts did not stop so many of my friends from shrugging it off and leaving me to crawl out of my despair alone.

When I looked up from the proverbial war zone that was my life at the time, I saw just a few remaining soldiers. These were the true friends that I clung to for dear life so that I could try to recover. They saved me, and they know who they are. One of them is my friend Kelly, and I will forever be grateful to her for seeing this for what it was and helping me make this book a reality. There are few gifts you get on the other side of this toxic relationship, but true friendships are one of the most tremendous among them. These are the friends who celebrate your boundaries, who honor your journey and will never shame you or victim-blame you for what you have endured. They revel in your ability to overcome this experience and will show up for you in a way that is validating and genuine.

You will lose childhood friends, family members, neighbors, and more, but you will gain a tribe of trusted confidants. Your circle may get smaller, but it will be sturdier and far safer than it was before. It ends up being a blessing when you see who can withstand the smear campaign and still love you for you. You deserve to love yourself and be loved by others, but having survived this horrible chapter of your life, you will now be more discerning in your selection of friends and partners. If they weren't so awful, you may have gratitude to the narcissist for giving you this gift.

THERAPY TIP: DEALING WITH THE FALL-OUT OF A SMEAR CAMPAIGN

As with everything else in dealing with a narcissist, this isn't easy, but there are some tips for dealing with the fallout of a narcissistic smear campaign.

- **Don't give them any attention.** As difficult as it may seem, staying calm and collected when dealing with a narcissist is essential. Sometimes, if someone refuses to react, this can help stop a smear campaign in its tracks. Alternatively, it may prompt the narcissist to become reactive, so that they reveal themselves to be the true abuser.

- **Only try to persuade true friends.** This can be one of the most frustrating things for victims of a narcissistic smear campaign. Unfortunately, trying to persuade the wrong person that the information they're being fed is false can have the opposite effect, making *you* look like the vindictive one. Those who believe a narcissist's lies are likely not your true friends.

- **Pick your battles.** If the narcissist is messing with your livelihood, family relationships, or children, you must address these issues, but if they are talking about stupid things or making wild accusations for which they have no proof, simply ignore their histrionics. It may take a long time, but eventually, their lies will catch up to them and their vindictive behaviors will shine through.

- **Stay connected to your support system.** This is essential to your healing and to spreading the truth. Staying in contact with people who are still communicating with your abuser is not recommended. You will need to lean on friends and family who are not part of the narcissist's attempts at triangulation.

- **Go "no-contact" or "low-contact."** If you are able to do so, going "no-contact" with the person who is smearing you is the best course of action. If you must have contact with them, only communicate with them when necessary regarding the children or any other business dealings. When you do, treat these interactions as exactly what they are: business transactions, no more, no less.

- **Tell a therapist.** Being the victim of a smear campaign can result in symptoms of depression and anxiety. A skilled therapist will help validate you and support you through these horrifying experiences. Although many therapists do not understand what this form of abuse is like for victims, there are some that do. See the Resources section, pages 275–277, to help you connect with therapists who can provide treatment for this specific kind of trauma. It's okay to ask them whether they have endured it themselves. I often share parts of my story through therapist self-disclosure (TSD) to validate my clients, and they report to me that they feel less crazy when I share tidbits and parallels with them.

Chapter 13

Trauma Bonding, Guilt, and Shame: The Cycle of Abuse

Connie came to me because she was feeling strong anxiety and couldn't sleep; she also wasn't sure what was happening with her partner, with whom she'd been for ten years. It took us a few sessions to really dig in. "Vanessa, I don't understand it. It's like we just keep doing this dance. He can be so . . . it's almost smothering, like, we have a huge blowout, and then he comes back, crying, saying how much he loves me, and I feel sorry for him. It's been ten years, after all, and I don't know; I'm not getting any younger; we have the house together, but his name is on the mortgage. What am I going to do, break up and move out of my own home? It's embarrassing and I don't think anyone would believe me if I told them about some of the stuff he does. . . ."

All the phases of an abusive relationship form a cycle, one that creates particularly dangerous and unhealthy attachments. Here, I synthesize everything we talked about so far in Part 2 and explore what these major phases of narcissistic abuse look like on the second go-round, when you may have had a falling-out and are "making up." This discussion warrants its own chapter because this is where the trauma bond—the victim's druglike attachment/addiction to the narcissist—develops. We will also unpack guilt and shame and how important it is for you to recognize and heal your shame to be able to move on.

The narcissistic cycle of abuse and violence is a pattern of behaviors that keeps you locked in the abusive relationship. This sequence of ups and downs creates a dynamic in which you are eager for the good or nice version of the narcissist to appear again, to the extent that you will work extremely hard to make that happen, sometimes sacrificing things you never thought you would in the process. Think of the ways a drug addict might rob their own children or parents to get their next fix. Similarly, and as we'll discuss further in Chapter 14, victims of narcissistic abuse will do the most shameful things because of their trauma bond with the narcissist. We see this in cults as well, where victims are asked to make statements harming their own reputation.

It is important to understand that these phases and the cycle that develops out of them are a standardized circle. This is sometimes called the "Groundhog Day phenomenon," after the 1993 film *Groundhog Day*, in which Bill Murray plays a TV weatherman who gets stuck in a time loop while covering the annual Groundhog Day event in Punxsutawney, Pennsylvania, forcing him to relive February 2 repeatedly. Narcissists will similarly repeat their harmful behaviors in a purposeful rhythm with just enough nuanced differences that you won't realize you're stuck in a pattern until it's too late. The rhythm and cyclical nature of their abuse is designed to be repetitive, so as to break you down and control you. Over time, through the narcissist's use of the cycle, they create so much confusion that it gives them the utmost control.

During the repetition of the cycle of abuse, the phases take on additional depth, highlighting three overarching phases that directly create the trauma bond between the narcissist and their supply: the makeup session phase, the tension-building phase, and the fight or falling-out phase. The corollaries are: the love-bombing (honeymoon/idealizing/makeup) phase, the devaluing (tension-building) phase, and the discard (fight/falling-out) phase often repeat in the cycle of abuse.

Cycle of Narcissist Abuse

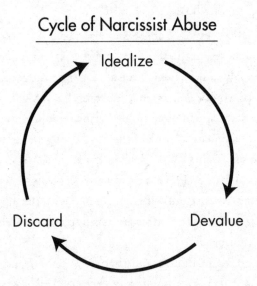

HOW REPETITION IMPACTS EACH PHASE IN THE CYCLE OF ABUSE

The narcissist's patterns of abuse are directed at almost everyone they engage with, often with very little change. You may even recall your storytelling narcissist repeating themselves over and over to you and others. The faces of their audience change, but the behaviors of the narcissist repeat.

To put it another way, their recurring and cyclical pattern of abuse is perpetuated by intermittent reinforcement through rewards and punishments. They bounce back and forth between the love-bombing phase and the mask-slipping phase, feigning remorse for each and every "unintended" slight or harm they enact against you.

Any relationship with a narcissist is therefore a weaponized series of dichotomies used to break the survivor down: loving and loathing, trust and distrust, distance and possession, and so on. This cycle of wounding and soothing, which we first talked about in Chapter 1, or reward and punishment, results in a survivor's neurological, psychological, and cognitive destabilization. As this progresses, the trauma and cognitive dissonance become stronger for the victim, and their communications with the narcissist become both crazier and more frequent, leading to more gaslighting and other traumatic forms of psychological abuse.

The Power and Control Wheel (detailed on the next page) is a particularly useful tool in understanding the overall pattern of abusive and violent behaviors that a narcissist uses to establish and maintain control over their partner. Very often, one or more violent incidents are accompanied by an array of these other types of abuse.

Love-Bombing → Makeup Stage

We have talked before about this early stage in the cycle of abuse. When we did, we called it the love-bombing stage because it was the first instance in which it happened. The mask had not yet slipped, and the charming narcissist was still seducing you.

Now, looking at subsequent turns of the cycle of abuse, we will refer to it as the "makeup" stage, meaning the period of time when a couple "makes up" after an argument. During the makeup stage, you are once again dazzled by the narcissist's gifts, compliments, and, with some narcissists, apologies. Sometimes, they will only have to give you breadcrumbs; sometimes even the removal of a punishment is enough! For instance, if the narcissist who has been purposely ignoring you sends you an innocuous text asking what days the recycling gets picked up, it will give you immense relief because they have broken the seemingly endless torture of the silent treatment. Many of my clients tell me that they become extremely agitated when the narcissist ignores them, to the extent that they will incessantly text and call them to get the coveted relief of not having to endure the silent

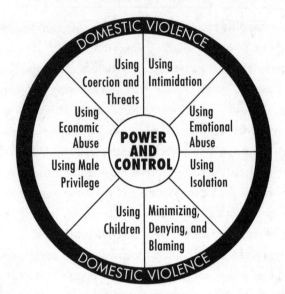

Using Intimidation
- Causing fear via dirty looks & threatening gestures
- Smashing things
- Abusing pets
- Displaying weapons

Using Emotional Abuse
- Using putdowns
- Devaluing/insulting
- Making victim feel crazy
- Playing mind games
- Humiliation
- Making victim feel guilty

Using Isolation
- Controlling what victim does
- Controlling who they see, talk to & what they read
- Controlling where they go
- Limiting outside involvement
- Using love to justify actions

Minimizing, Denying, and Blaming
- Making light of abuse
- Denying abuse happened
- Blame shifting

Using Children
- Making victim feel guilty about children
- Using children to relay messages
- Using visitation to harass victim
- Threatening to take children

Using Male Privilege
- Treating victim like a servant
- Acting like a master
- Defining all roles traditionally

Economic Abuse
- Preventing victim from getting or keeping a job
- Making victim ask for money
- Giving an allowance
- Taking/controlling victim's money
- Withholding financial information

Using Coercion and Threats
- Making and/or carrying out threats to do something to hurt the victim
- Threatening to leave the victim
- Threatening to commit suicide
- Threatening to take children away
- Making them do illegal things

treatment any longer. The removal of the love-bombing positive reinforcer is enough to cause many victims to spiral into self-doubt and wonder what they are doing wrong.

You will ultimately yearn for this part of the cycle because it is where the abuser appears to feel remorse for the emotional, psychological, physical, verbal, or sexual abuse that they have caused. They may promise through tears, or with what appears to be a sincere apology, that they will never do it again. In most situations, you believe them, even when it has happened a handful of times before, because you *want* to believe them. The abuser may even push the blame onto you at this point, telling you that they were forced to respond the way that they did. Had you not acted in a certain way or said the wrong things, you would never have been abused the way that you were. The narcissist may also gaslight you, telling you that the abuse never took place or that you are exaggerating the severity of the incident. You may start to realize that the narcissist is all sizzle and no steak. They are as if "clickbait" were a person.

Mask-Slipping / Devaluation → Tension-Building Stage

This time through the cycle, the narcissist has started to exhibit some of the same patterns they just apologized for, but they may up the ante.

When the makeup stage is followed by the tension-building stage, trauma bonding occurs. I explain trauma bonding in more detail in Chapter 14, but in short, it is when you become addicted to your abuser fixing things as well as the making up in the relationship. The narcissist will then start dropping subtle hints that you've done something wrong and may be passive-aggressive or give you that dreaded silent treatment. You'll start to feel insecure and wonder why they told you that they would change when they have made no efforts to do so. You will likely feel riddled with shame when this stage repeatedly shows up; you believed them the first time they said they would not behave badly again, but now, this is the encore.

As a result, the tension-building stage can leave you feeling depressed, anxious, confused, and scared of losing your relationship with the narcissist. You might either try harder to please them or pull away from them to protect yourself. If you choose the latter, the narcissist will feel hurt and enraged by your attempts to distance yourself from them, which can become dangerous. You may feel that you need to be very careful with any words that you speak; my clients often describe themselves as "walking on eggshells" during this phase.

NARCISSISTIC ABUSE AND SHAME

Shame is the primary tool used by abusers to cow their victims. They pass judgments and create feelings of shame, especially in this devaluing or tension-building stage of the cycle of abuse. Identifying the sources of your shame and judgment is instrumental, not only in healing and breaking away from the cycle of abuse, but also in living a healthier life. Coming to understand how shame works to diminish you is the very first step toward escaping from an emotionally abusive relationship, so let's get into it.

Shame at the hands of a narcissist happens covertly, quietly, and stealthily at first. It begins as the occasional subtle dig but grows over time as the narcissist is able to gauge what you will endure. They may ask you if you are "really going to eat that" or "where do you think you are going dressed like that." Many victims hide the fact that they are being abused from their family and friends, due to this omnipresent shame, and yet keeping this secret creates even more shame. Some victims will even decide to leave their career, home, and friends behind, only furthering their level of shame by deciding to stay with someone who treats them terribly. In time, the walls of the prison of shame seem to close in around you as the distance between you and those who truly care most about you grows.

In this way, shame slowly deteriorates your self-esteem and confidence, and eventually makes you question your perception of reality. Victims of narcissistic abuse who are experiencing shame will feel incompetent, worthless, or otherwise "in need" of their abuser. Regrettably, once these shame-related feelings set in, you will become worn down, weakened, and confused, and will lose your ability to fight back.

The effects of shame from tolerating a narcissist's attacks are many, and they include:

- Self-hatred
- Self-harm
- Self-neglect (e.g., starving yourself, depriving yourself of proper nutrition, not practicing good hygiene)
- Substance abuse
- Anger
- Isolation
- Sunken body posture
- Blushing cheeks
- Increased body temperature
- Sweating
- Nausea

To gain the courage, strength, and determination to end an emotionally abusive relationship with a narcissist, survivors first need to rid themselves of their shame, but this can be easier said than done. Shame is, by far, the most destructive aspect of emotional abuse, and it can be the most difficult to heal. This is because it causes victims to stay and endure what they are convinced they deserve. You may start to believe that this abusive relationship is the best you can do and that you will never experience anything better than it.

When you are consistently shamed, you come to feel you are worthless and unlovable, especially if you had an abusive parent or caregiver growing up, because the narcissistically abusive relationship you've become trapped in as an adult only reinforces your preexisting beliefs.

But it is important to understand that **there is categorically no shame in having fallen for a narcissist.** These people are slick storytellers with the gift of gab, who could sell a ketchup ice pop to a woman in a white dress. Some people think that the narcissist only goes after people who are vulnerable or unintelligent. That is unequivocally untrue. Take, for instance, Felicia Rosario, a smart, successful, Harvard- and Columbia University–trained young physician who was brainwashed into Lawrence "Larry" Ray's sex trafficking cult at Sarah Lawrence College (depicted in the documentary *Stolen Youth*)—all the way from Los Angeles where she was completing her residency in forensic psychiatry! There are countless stories of highly intelligent people falling for manipulations of a narcissistic person.

Victims of emotional abuse also come from a wide range of age, race, level of socioeconomic status, gender, and sexual identity. It simply does not matter how smart you are, how powerful you are, or how much money you have. You were not stupid or naive for becoming attracted to an abusive person. Most abusers present themselves as caring, emotionally healthy individuals, not the shame-inducing, controlling, manipulative people they turn out to be. So, please stop blaming yourself for not seeing through their facade or not recognizing the abusive side to your partner. You don't know what you don't know.

You also should not blame yourself for not walking away at the first signs of abuse. After all, you likely loved your partner, and you wanted to give them the benefit of the doubt. You wanted to believe their promises when they said they would never treat you like that again.

Victims of emotional abuse tend to minimize their partner's abusive behavior and the effect it is having on them because they see it as "less harmful" than other, more physical forms of abuse. They are often the ones who will try to make excuses to their friends and family about their toxic partner's bad behavior. Maybe you can relate. Maybe, in spite of the fact that your partner's abusive behavior was escalating, you assured yourself and others that it wasn't that bad. Perhaps you heard stories of intimate partner abuse or domestic violence, and considered your experience to be altogether different because your partner was not physically abusive, but this is not the case. Remember what we discussed about the long-term, post-traumatic effects of narcissistic abuse? While the scars may not be visible, the trauma is real.

The shame we feel about being in an emotionally abusive relationship can be worsened by the reactions of others outside the relationship. This is because victims of emotional abuse are often criticized for not standing up for themselves when their partner first became abusive, or for not leaving sooner "if it was so bad"—a highly damaging form of victim blaming. Victim blaming is oftentimes perpetuated by the very people and organizations that are supposed to be there to believe us and protect us. It is not you. This is a common staple for survivors to experience and it is ultra-important to remove yourself from those environments as much as you can. In the case of the judicial system victim blaming, we have much work to do to change the system to include more trauma-informed practices.

Nowhere is the shame of being in a relationship with a narcissist or a cult more marked to clinicians than when their therapy client faces cajoling from their family members to leave, or at least see that they are in a toxic relationship and need to get out. Many family members, sensing the urgency of the situation, make the mistake of shaming their loved ones further, and this does nothing but push them back into the cult or relationship. [A note to anyone who loves a victim of narcissistic abuse who might be reading this: *Please* watch your tone when you're trying to communicate with a loved one who is stuck in this misery. Understand that they are already walking on eggshells and so ashamed of what they have been willing to tolerate. Hold space for them and do everything you can to be a safe place to land. Try talking to them about who they used to be. You might even get creative, using the five senses, such as cooking them their favorite meal or sending them a link to an old favorite song, to encourage their subconscious to return to the safe, loving relationships in their life.]

While some family members and friends do succeed at being a safe place to land, most people do not understand that abusers are very adept at handling the concerns voiced by their partners. Each time you noticed something you didn't like about the way your abuser was treating you, they may have passed it off as your being too critical. They may have listened to your concerns and apologized profusely, so as to rein you back in, but each time you forgave them and they failed or disappointed you, your shame increased. As you realized that the troubling behavior was not going away and was actually getting worse, your partner may have started to convince you that these kinds of problems are "normal" for couples to experience or that they are your fault. Many people will simply comply with the narcissist to avoid the name-calling, stonewalling, gaslighting, and passive aggression—in other words, the further shame—that comes from calling them out.

Unless you recognize your shame and begin to heal its wounds, your hands will feel tied, in terms of being unable to escape the relationship. Shame will cause you to curl up and feel smaller at a time when you need to stand up and feel empowered. It will cause you to blame yourself for your partner's actions and to feel badly about how you have reacted to their abuse. To gain the courage, strength, and determination to confront an abuser and/or end an emotionally abusive relationship, victims need to rid themselves of their shame. We will discuss some means of recognizing and beginning to heal shame, both in the Therapy Tip at the end of this chapter and in Chapter 17. By focusing on healing your shame, you will begin to believe in yourself and in your right to be happy and have autonomy. It is virtually impossible to heal in the place where you are being abused and therefore wounded, so when you become empowered to reject shame, you can begin to work toward getting away from your abuser and then focus on further healing.

THE DIFFERENCE BETWEEN SHAME AND GUILT

You may have noticed that I didn't use the word "guilt" at all in the previous section, and this was very much on purpose. The two emotions of shame and guilt are often confused with each other, but for our purposes, and in a therapeutic setting, guilt and shame are very different.

Guilt, it may surprise you to learn, can be healthy. It can keep you on track when you've drifted from your moral standards and is something that actually indicates empathy, so we are *healthy* if we have this experience from time to time. *Guilt* is an internal response to something you have done or something you haven't done, often something that goes against your ethics or fundamental values. You can often fix or repair something that you feel guilty about, but even if you can't repair it directly, changing your behavior or paying the reparation forward can alleviate guilt. People who are experiencing shame, meanwhile, are unable to see themselves separate from the act or infraction. *Shame* is a painful sense of being fundamentally bad. Guilt tells you, "That thing you did was bad," but shame tells you, "Because you did that thing, you're a bad person." For example, if you offended a friend, guilt would prompt you to apologize and repair the mistake. Shame, on the other hand, might cause you to spiral because you think that unintentionally offending that friend makes you a bad person.

The shame that comes from the repeated cycle of narcissistic abuse is fundamentally *different*. You feel shame when you believe you're not enough, usually because a toxic person, such as a narcissistic partner, parent, or friend, keeps sending you messages that this is so. Your confidence can suffer from this, and so, even outside of abusive relationships, we need to learn to stop shaming others through passive aggression and sarcasm, and we need to stop letting others shame us just as casually. Be mindful of people in your life who are dishing out silent jabs because this can affect your overall well-being.

––––⊗⊗⊗–––

In his book *The Culture of Shame*, Harvard psychiatric professor Dr. Andrew Morrison writes that shame feels like a weight that presses us down emotionally and physically and makes us want to "sink into the ground," disappear, or become invisible, simply because it makes us feel inferior, incompetent, and generally bad. It is accompanied by feelings of self-criticism and fear of being criticized by others.[1]

We cannot atone for or fix shame because, even when it's focused on something specific, such as our appearance or our failings, shame colors our whole identity and therefore our presence in the world. The narcissist will use this against you, shaming you over and over again until this sense of self-doubt and lack of worth becomes your everyday baseline.

When you instead take responsibility for your actions without beating yourself up, you can combat shame and then develop a sense of agency, power, and strength, which can help counter further feelings of defectiveness and inadequacy. This is critically important to escape from the narcissistic cult of one or cult of many, for only by healing your sense of shame can you begin to move on. The combination of taking genuine responsibility and making reparations for things you have done can be a powerful way to fight shame. It is my hope that the lessons in the remaining chapters of this book will help you do just that.

THERAPY TIP: PRACTICE LESS JUDGMENT

We all have negative feelings and bad days from time to time, so the idea behind this tip is to try to rewrite, in our mind, our negative feelings into a form that is entirely nonjudgmental. This nonjudgmental stance, as described in dialectical behavioral therapy (DBT), refers to the ability to judge circumstances, people, behaviors, and experiences as neither good nor bad, and to focus simply on the facts at hand. This shift in your thinking and perspective will teach you how to express a negative thought without the "judgy" attitude that often comes with it. It is an exercise in logical thinking without any fatalistic thoughts that can contribute to negative self-esteem or self-worth.

Judgment of others, ourselves, and our experiences is a way of trying to enforce our preferences and wants, most often in situations we can't control, and are mostly instinctual. The problem is, we sometimes forget that our judgments are not facts but are our preferences and opinions based on our own experiences. When we are particularly stressed, we are more likely to think judgmentally and use an inner dialogue that includes such words as: "unfair," "shouldn't," "stupid," "bad," "terrible," and "wrong." Judgmental thinking can often get us in trouble.

The challenge is the spontaneity of our judgments and thoughts. Forming judgments is a reflexive mental process, and there are times when we need to make judgments to keep out of harm's way, but to reduce emotional reactivity in everyday situations, it's important to become aware of our own judgmental thinking and to develop the ability to think nonjudgmentally. This skill is so important for people to understand and practice, so that we can all live in a world that works toward practicing empathy, not just toward others, but toward ourselves!

To do this, we need to step back and interrupt the process by mindfully considering our emotions and what is prompting them rather than focusing on the thing or person on which we are tempted to pass judgment. This is the first step in reducing our emotional reactivity when things don't go our way. Learning to objectively describe our emotions and the situation at hand can help us slow down, calm down, and take back control.

As with many things in life, achieving a nonjudgmental mental framework comes with practice. Try to think about something that you are judging as you go throughout your day, and then describe the situation factually. Write down the feeling you had and what you were thinking about that prompted that feeling. The following are three examples to get you started.

Example 1

Observation: I notice that I am angry at something my partner did/said.

Description: I notice that my brow is in a scowl, I feel shaky, and my muscles are tense.

Judgment: Anger is a bad emotion. Anger means I'm bad. Something is wrong with me because I feel angry.

Nonjudgmental Stance: Anger is a normal emotion. It is neither good nor bad. Being angry doesn't mean I'm a bad person, and experiencing anger isn't a good or bad thing. It is okay to be angry, and I have control over how I exhibit my anger.

Possible Results: When I judge my anger, I am more likely to react in a negative way and to be destructive in my relationships. When I avoid judging my anger, I am more

likely to acknowledge it and experience it until it goes
away, without harming myself or the people I love.

Example 2

Observation: I notice I am annoyed at this driver in front of
me, who is going too slow in the fast lane.

Description: I notice I am tense, and my neck and chest are
tight. My eyes feel heavy, and I feel on edge.

Judgment: This stupid driver isn't paying attention and
doesn't know how to drive. They are annoying me
and shouldn't be on the road. I hate that I'm annoyed and
irritated; I don't want to feel this way. I am going to be
late because of this jerk.

Nonjudgmental Stance: Being annoyed makes sense in
this present situation. That person is driving slow in the
wrong lane, which makes me feel unsafe. The situation
has triggered annoyance and irritation, which is a normal
reaction.

Possible Results: When I fight my annoyance or irritation
and deem it as bad, I am more likely to react negatively
or impulsively. When I avoid judging my annoyance, I'm
more likely to remain annoyed for a short amount of time
without driving recklessly or lashing out. As a result, I'm
also more likely to arrive at my destination safely.

Chapter 14

Why We Stay— The Trauma Bond

After Rebecca escaped from her abuser, she kept waiting for him to show up and "fix" it. In a session, she said she shook for a week like a drug addict going through withdrawal—she needed that "fix." She said the end result of freedom was worth it, but the pain was excruciating as she went through her "narcissist detox."

---

he discussion of the trauma bond you'll find in this chapter is very important because it describes what biologically occurs when you get swept up in a relationship with a narcissist, a phenomenon very similar to that of a drug addiction, as my client Rebecca noted.

If you have ever asked yourself or anyone else, "If they were so awful to you, why did you stay?" this chapter will help you understand the biochemical experience of the trauma bond; what a healthy attachment looks like versus an unhealthy attachment; scenarios and syndromes similar to trauma bonding; and even what a trauma bond is not.

WHAT IS A TRAUMA BOND?

The term *trauma bond* describes how feelings of fear, excitement, and sex can manipulate, trap, or entangle another person. Periods of intense love and excitement followed by episodes of abuse, neglect, and mistreatment create a corrupt attachment, through intermittent reinforcement in the cycle of abuse, to an abusive person. There are enough good days to entice you, enough bad days to confuse you, and enough enablers to put forth their fake persona. These patterns of being devalued and then rewarded repeatedly create a strong hormonal bond between you and your abuser. As we'll discuss later in this chapter, experiencing such trauma as a child could make you more prone to developing these types of relationships as an adult because you associate this kind of behavior with the caregivers you had in early life. Therefore, your nervous system might already be prepped to continue these patterns and cycles. The shorter the length of time between when they show their Jekyll and Hyde sides, the stronger the trauma bond. The longer the span between these ups and downs, the harder they are to detect and the longer the relationship, which is worse in many ways because it robs you of your most precious commodity: time.

LOVE CHEMICALS

When a person falls in love, they experience certain chemical reactions in the brain. A cocktail of different hormones, such as serotonin, vasopressin, norepinephrine, and dopamine, which have been proven to elicit a pleasurable experience similar to the euphoria associated with the use of cocaine, alcohol, nicotine, and amphetamines, is responsible for this feeling of glee when we experience a new love attachment. There are a variety of physical and emotional responses, such as a racing heartbeat, sweaty hands, flushed cheeks, and feelings of passion and anxiety that come with feeling new love. Levels of the stress hormone cortisol increase during the initial phase of romantic love, commissioning our body to cope with the "crisis" at hand.

Another combination of hormones at work during the early days of romantic love is oxytocin and vasopressin, which play positive roles in pregnancy, nursing, and mother-infant attachment. Released during sex and heightened by skin-to-skin contact, oxytocin deepens feelings of attachment and makes couples feel closer to each other by provoking feelings of contentment, calmness, and security. Vasopressin similarly is linked to behavior that produces long-term, monogamous relationships.

According to Richard Schwartz and Jacqueline Olds of Harvard Medical School, the differences in behavior associated with the actions of these two hormones may explain why passionate love fades as attachment grows—that is, as our attachment to another person feels stronger and more secure, we feel less cortisol-induced stress over our anxiety to keep them. Schwartz and Olds emphasize that love also deactivates the neural pathway responsible for negative emotions, such as fear and judgment.[1] This neurological pathway connects the nucleus accumbens, a tiny part of the brain that helps us link motivation to action, with the amygdala, a part of the brain that helps us learn and process emotions and memories. When we are engaged in romantic love, the neural machinery responsible for making critical assessments, including assessments of those with whom we are romantically involved, shuts down. "That's the neural basis for the ancient wisdom 'love is blind,'" says Schwartz.[2] We generally have heightened emotions and passionate feelings for one to two years at the start of a relationship, and then we continue to have the passion, but the stress of it is gone. Cortisol and serotonin levels return to normal. Love, which began as a stressor, becomes a buffer *against* stress.

The chemicals at the beginning of all love affairs are the same. When you are in an abusive relationship, you do not get these benefits of being in love, but the brain and body do not know the difference. According to biological anthropologist Dr. Helen Fisher, "the brains of those in adversity-ridden relationships become activated in an eerily similar way to the brains of cocaine addicts."[3]

SIGNS OF TRAUMA BONDING

Some people mistakenly believe a trauma bond is when two people share a deep connection over past trauma that they have experienced, either together or separately. In some cases, this type of bonding could be positive and is therefore *not* defined as a "trauma bond," which takes place exclusively in abusive relationships.

A trauma bond actually develops when narcissistic abusers use coercive control to make you believe you need the abuser's care and validation to feel sufficient. You become highly dependent on the abusive relationship, whether it be romantic or family-, friend-, or work-related. Humans form attachments as a means of survival. Babies become attached to the caregivers upon whom they depend, and adults form attachments to others who provide comfort and support, but these are not attachment issues. A trauma bond, in contrast, is orchestrated effort by someone to make you believe that they are your guardian and protector, only for them to pull out the rug from under you. You may rely on the person causing you the pain to be the one who rescues you from it. In the case of an abusive parent, the child may come to associate love with abuse, believing that this association is normal, and become unable to see what is happening to them. This allows the caregiver to continue being "good" in the child's eyes, which reinforces their bond.

Trauma bonding has similarities to capture-bonding, also known as Stockholm syndrome, a psychological phenomenon in which people who are being held captive develop feelings of trust and affection toward their captors and begin to identify closely with their agenda and demands. The name of the syndrome is derived from a botched robbery that took place in Stockholm, Sweden, in August 1973, in which four employees of Sveriges Kreditbank were held hostage in the bank's vault for six days. During the standoff, a seemingly contradictory bond developed between captive and captor, and the hostages expressed more fear of the police than of the people holding them hostage.[4]

The most infamous example of Stockholm syndrome may be that involving kidnapped newspaper heiress Patty Hearst in 1974. Some ten weeks after being taken hostage by the Symbionese Liberation Army, Hearst helped her kidnappers rob a California bank.

Psychologists who have studied Stockholm syndrome believe that the bond is initially created when a captor threatens a captive's life, deliberates, and then chooses not to kill the captive. The captive's relief at the removal of the death threat is transferred into feelings of gratitude toward the captor. In this way, it is not dissimilar to the trauma bond. The person who experiences the trauma bond as a result of the cycle of abuse will consider the removal of any punishment, whether passive aggression, the silent treatment, or even physical abuse, similarly. In other words, just by virtue of the fact that the abuser *stops* punishing you, you feel both relieved and bonded to them. It is a reward, of sorts; a negative reinforcement. As the Stockholm bank robbery illustrates, it takes only a few days for this bond to cement, proving that, early on, the victim's desire to survive trumps their urge to hate the person who created the situation.

In many cases, the only difference between Stockholm syndrome and the trauma bond is the victim's level of fear for their life. In both cases, victims live in a state of enforced dependence and interpret rare or small acts of kindness in the midst of horrible conditions as good treatment. They often become hypervigilant to the needs and demands of their captors/abusers, making psychological links between the captors' happiness and their own. Many victims of abuse will begin to feel that if they try harder or show more affection, things will be fine. If you do manage to break free from the trauma bond, the abuser will commonly revert to the courtship phase to win you back, which works more often than not. Indeed, the two disordered attachments are marked, not only by a positive bond between captive/abusee and captor/abuser, but also by the captive/abusee's negative attitude toward authorities or friends who threaten the captor-captive relationship.

Along with hostages and victims of narcissistic abuse, prisoners of war, procured prostitutes, and victims of human trafficking—and cult members—often suffer similar experiences. *Trauma, fear, and abandonment actually increase feelings of attachment, so the more you have been hurt by a narcissistic cult leader, the more intensely attached to them you will be.*

It is worth noting that these feelings of attachment do not necessarily end when a person leaves a harmful situation. A person may still feel loyal or loving toward the person who abused them or may feel tempted to return to their side. If you want to leave someone, but you can't bring yourself to cut them out of your life, you may have a trauma bond. You might even decide it is best for your overall health to leave this person, but the impetus to go back to them is so powerful that you lose your resolve.

Please understand that, as a survivor of narcissistic abuse, it is highly unlikely that your relationship with your abuser will ever get back to the love-bombing phase or the initial high of being with the charming and manipulative narcissist. When you justify the abusive behavior in a toxic relationship, you are only creating a skewed narrative of the situation that not only encourages this kind of behavior but causes you to build a wall around the root of the problem. This wall is built out of fear of what might happen if you don't accept all the ugliness of the abusive relationship.

INTERMITTENT REINFORCEMENT

When you go through the cycle of abuse repeatedly, you will develop an addiction to the highs you experienced in the love-bombing and makeup stages of the relationship. As indicated earlier in this chapter, victims of the cycle of abuse become so addicted to these good moments that they are willing to ignore the destructive phases that prevent a healthy, loving emotional connection from ever forming. Clients express to me that trauma bonding makes it feel as though the only person who can fix their pain is the abuser—the one who actually caused it. This is the same way that a drug addict feels.

This addiction happens through a process called *intermittent reinforcement*. Intermittent reinforcement is the delivery of a reward at irregular intervals, and it becomes standard in trauma-bonded relationships. In fact, trauma bonding happens specifically because an abuser provides you with intermittent rewards and punishments. In doing so, a psychological conditioning takes place, whereby the survivor becomes entangled in the relationship, always hoping to return to the "when it's good, it's good" time frame. Eventually, you will settle for almost any little breadcrumb of the version of who the narcissist was in the beginning. You may even settle for not being punished as a reward, or for a version of love-bombing.

At this point in the relationship, victims of abuse are so emotionally starved that the "reward" their abuser gives them actually triggers their brain's reward center, which then floods the parts of the brain that produce and deliver dopamine, as well as stimulates the hypothalamus, which aims to keep your body in an internally balanced state. The victim will have such an intense craving for the "reward" when they don't have it, that they'll lose sight and control of themselves in pursuit of it. They'll remain trauma-bonded to the relationship, despite its negative consequences on their mental and physical health because the "reward" they randomly receive from their abuser has become their only known source of happiness. After all, every other thing that may have brought them happiness— such as their friends, family, career, and hobbies—has been systematically removed from their grasp.

What people need to understand is that victims of narcissistic abuse are drawn back into these situations because they are effectively "love junkies." Just like someone who struggles with heroin withdrawal, the victim of narcissistic abuse will obsessively think about how to get back to that "happy" place in the relationship. They think that if they can only "use" one more time, they'll feel better about themselves, but they don't.

If you've been through this situation, then you know how it is to think that if you can just talk to your abuser one more time, if you can go through their social media, or if you can see them and try to reason with them, it'll make you feel better. I cannot tell you how many clients I have that are stuck in this loop. They spend countless hours trying to explain to their abuser what they should be doing differently, and hey, I was no different. This can go on for a lifetime! People blame themselves and feel so much shame around staying close to their addiction, and unfortunately, this isn't always clear to their family and friends. Just like the family and friends of a drug abuser, they might say to you, "Why do you keep going back to this person who's treating you so terribly?" It doesn't make sense to them.

ATTACHMENT STYLES

Narcissistic relationships trap us in a perpetual, traumatic cycle of tension, abuse, and reconciliation that ties us closer to our abusers, one orbit at a time. If you had a tumultuous childhood, this cycle can feel almost comforting because it's all you've ever known. The tumult *itself* is mistaken for fervor and passion while a healthy relationship, which lacks this turbulence, can feel flat in comparison.

Nearly everyone feels an attachment to someone. You may have an attachment to one or more of your parents, or you may feel particularly close to an extended family member or friend. If you have children or a romantic partner, you likely have an attachment to them, and you might even feel the same way about a coworker. Understanding the many types of attachment styles will help us comprehend the difference between a healthy attachment and the trauma bond; it will also help us understand what different attachment styles mean for the victims and survivors of narcissistic abuse.

Researchers have studied attachment styles for many decades. In the mid-twentieth century, psychoanalyst John Bowlby developed his own attachment theory. Bowlby's work was primarily with children and adolescents, but he acknowledged that attachments form throughout the life span. Mary Ainsworth, an associate of Bowlby's, developed theories about infant attachment, and later on, Cindy Hazan and Phillip Shaver used Bowlby's and Ainsworth's concepts to develop adult attachment theory.

Here are the main types of attachment styles:

- Secure
- Anxious
- Avoidant
- Disorganized

Secure Attachment

The origin of **secure attachment** comes from Ainsworth's "strange situation" test, which explored an infant's relationship to their parent or caregiver. An infant with secure attachment explored freely when the caregiver was nearby. Whenever the infant felt distressed, they would come close to the caregiver for reassurance; then, they would go back to exploring. When the caregiver left, the infant showed only mild distress. When the caregiver returned, the infant quickly reestablished contact.

A secure attachment provides many benefits to the developing child, including:

- Enhanced learning
- Healthy physical, emotional, intellectual, and social development
- Curiosity
- Being more outgoing
- An ability to explore their environment freely
- Less aggression
- More empathy
- More creativity
- More persistence
- An ability to cope with difficulties more easily
- A greater ability to form a social network
- Being better at choosing romantic partners

An adult who is empathetic and able to set appropriate boundaries has a secure attachment style. People with secure attachment tend to feel safer, more stable, and more satisfied in their close relationships, and while they don't fear being on their own, they usually thrive in close, meaningful relationships.

Adults with a secure attachment style possess these characteristics:

- A positive view of themselves
- A healthy balance of being self-sufficient and being comfortable asking for support when they need it
- The ability to trust others
- A joy to be around

- The capacity to develop and maintain strong relationships
- Emotional balance
- The ability to emotionally regulate people close to them

Anxious Attachment

When you have an **anxious attachment**, you may feel that your life is difficult, and you may suffer from anxiety, depression, or other mental health challenges. Your romantic, social, and professional relationships may be volatile if your unhealthy attachment style keeps you from connecting in a positive way with your partner, friends, or coworkers.

The development of an anxious attachment style may come from a lack of trust and a lack of a secure base, due to early separation from a parent or caregiver, a troubled childhood, including physical or sexual abuse and instances of neglect or mistreatment. When adults with a secure attachment look back on their childhood, they usually feel that someone reliable was always available to them, whereas people with an anxious attachment style may have felt neglected or unseen. People with an anxious attachment style may behave in anxious, ambivalent, or unpredictable ways, including being mistrusting of others and intensely afraid of abandonment. You can heal from anxious attachment by understanding what it is and where it originates from, spending time with people with secure attachment, building your self-esteem, practicing expressing your emotional needs, learning to not react, and of course, my favorite: therapy.

Adults with anxious attachment possess these characteristics:

- Intense emotional discomfort or avoidance of being alone
- Difficulty setting boundaries[5]
- Fear of abandonment[6]
- Feeling unworthy of love
- Feeling dependent on others
- Frequent need for validation
- Sensitivity to changes in how others feel, speak, or behave
- Tolerating unhealthy behaviors in relationships
- Difficulty trusting others

Avoidant Attachment

Avoidant attachment is an insecure attachment style marked by fear and indifference, brought on in children by a parent or caregiver who is consistently emotionally unavailable or unresponsive to their needs. Infants with an avoidant attachment style may also have faced repeated discouragement from crying or expressing outward emotion. In the "strange situation" test, infants with this attachment style didn't explore much when their caregiver was present, and when their caregiver left and returned, they showed no signs that they noticed their absence. Some even avoided their caregiver altogether when they returned.

Infants with an avoidant attachment style may learn not to seek help or comfort because their primary caregiver has failed to provide them with these benefits. They have learned that the best way to stay close to their caregiver is to hide those feelings. As they age, they may develop a critical inner voice that tells them to avoid people, not to get involved, and not to invest in romantic relationships, much less trust people. The characteristics of adult avoidant attachment style include:

* Not relying on others
* Not expressing needs
* Having difficulty maintaining intimate relationships
* Struggling with conflict and vulnerability
* Being turned off by clingy partners[7]

These are people who dissociate from the concept of needing social interactions to survive and who will avoid intimacy in most situations. People with avoidant attachment can heal by understanding what it is and where it originates from, spending time with people with secure attachment, cultivating healthy communication, challenging self-critical thoughts, and therapy.

Disorganized Attachment/Anxious Avoidant

Brought on by fear-arousing behaviors, or confusing and conflicting communication in a child's parent, **disorganized or anxious avoidant**

attachment styles are when you may not know quite how to feel about your partner. You might seek their help at one moment, ignore them the next, and fight with them later. Relationships can be volatile when you have a disorganized attachment style. You might want to stay in some relationships, but you may ultimately drive your partner away with your unpredictability. It can also be hard to keep a job or advance your career when no one knows what to expect from you.

People with disorganized attachment often exhibit:

- Dismissive attitudes
- Little interest in relationships
- Avoidance of intimacy
- Limited ability to reach out or connect with others[8]

While it can be helpful to explore your own attachment style, it is important to disconnect attachment styles from narcissistic abuse, because people who have an unhealthy attachment style *and* an interest in working on it are likely not narcissists *at all*. In other words, *do not* make the unhealthy assumption that the abuser in your life just has an issue with attachment and that it can be fixed. If that is not true, you may find yourself with a huge problem. Abusers may use excuses around attachment styles to avoid accountability, but someone with an issue with their attachment style can definitely seek help from a skilled professional to work on developing more secure attachments.

Some ways to develop a more secure attachment include the following.

- Seek out others with secure attachment styles.
- Learn about your attachment style.
- Examine your beliefs about relationships.
- Act opposite to your anxious or avoidant style.
- Increase your emotional awareness.
- Communicate openly and listen empathetically.[9]

BREAKING THE TRAUMA BOND

Still unsure as to whether you're experiencing a trauma bond? Ask yourself the following questions:

- Would you ever want your friends, family, or peers to be in the same kind of relationship?
- Does your situation look toxic when you visualize another person in the same predicament?
- Do you have to keep repeating that others don't understand your relationship?
- Do you often find yourself "selling" or "pitching" the good parts of the narcissist to others? You may be working tirelessly to fix the narcissist's reputation all whilst he is wrecking yours.
- Does this person have characteristics that remind you of a toxic parent or caregiver?
- Do you know it is best to leave, but you simply cannot make the moves to do so?
- Do you feel confused or afraid if you are apart from them?

Answering these questions for yourself can lend insight into the reality of how you are living in this relationship. If you cannot justify what you're going through, much less wish that a friend, family member, or peer were going through it, too, then not only are you developing a trauma bond, but you would benefit from seeking help and support from professionals. Much like kicking a drug habit, there are going to be powerful withdrawals once you've broken the addictive component of a trauma bond. A therapist that understands narcissistic abuse is going to be able to help you work through those withdrawals and give you the information needed to ensure that you don't find yourself back in the abuse cycle.

Additionally, the addictive component is only one reason that breaking a trauma bond can be so challenging. By diving into the hidden aspects of trauma bonding with a trained professional, you may uncover the people pleasing, approval seeking, or codependency in childhood that primed you for this.

Further, just because you've broken a trauma bond doesn't mean that the trauma has gone with it. Taking the time to learn how to conceptualize a realistic sense of self without the abuser is going to help you find the healthy, happy, and secure environment that you deserve. (See Resources, pages 275–277, for links to info on how to find a therapist.)

THERAPY TIP: TWO LISTS

Here are two things that helped me break the trauma bond for myself and that I now always counsel my clients to do:

1. **Make a list of all the bad things the narcissist has done to you.** Make this list robust and fluid. Keep it handy in your cell phone so you can look at it and add to it as you remember things. This list is to help with cognitive dissonance when you forget what you have endured. Should you become triggered, take a break and try to "microdose" your exposure. In other words, if it becomes too heavy, do it in increments.

2. **Make a list of things that you love about yourself.** Make sure these things are not contingent upon how others experience you. It should be things like being smart or funny, not kind or giving, because while those personal attributes are great, they are dependent on the approval of others. This list is designed to get you to practice radical self-love and to step into your power, something the narcissist is allergic to. In some ways, you are going to feel selfish in developing this list. If you have a hard time developing this list—and many people pleasers

do—commission trusted friends and family members who are good cheerleaders to help you. It can be such a treat to hear from them just how wonderful you are.

Some clients have told me that they are:
- Creative
- Smart
- Strong
- Funny
- Curious

Chapter 15

"I Believe You!"—
Domestic Violence

When I got away from my abusive ex, it was at times an uphill battle to determine who was in my corner. At the time I was on the board of a domestic violence (DV) center and friendly with other board members, and I thought I could turn to them for advice.

In the aftermath of my escape, I was reeling, even wondering, thanks to the way my ex had mirrored me so adeptly, whether I was the abuser. I needed my colleagues' trusted guidance. I will never forget what one board member said to me when I confided in her: "We believe both of you." It was so hurtful to feel disbelieved by the one entity that was put in place to validate me and believe me. I suspected, at that moment, that my ex's large donations to the center over the years may have influenced their opinion. In retrospect, it felt like the personal equivalent of Trump's 2017 press conference when he talked about the protest in Charlottesville, Virginia, as having "very fine people on both sides."

T here are not two sides of the story when it comes to abuse. There are the abuser's lies and the truth. This has been one of the hardest parts of my journey to healing—the people that were supposed to be there for me were not; they ultimately asked me to remain quiet about what I had endured. I refuse to be silent about it.

I introduced the relationship between domestic violence and narcissism in Chapter 1; in this chapter, I cover what we all need to know about it. But first, an important reminder.

POSTSEPARATION ABUSE

The level of vindictiveness in this part of the narcissistic relationship can be sociopathic in nature, possibly to a tragic level. When a relationship with a narcissist ends, there are a lot of ways that the narcissist might harm their victims within and outside of the smear campaign.

Here are some other ways the narcissist may perpetrate postseparation abuse.

- **Isolation:** The narcissist works overtime to assassinate their victims' reputation. This might include cyber-gaslighting them on social media so that friends, family, colleagues, and congregations will subscribe to the idea of their "losing it" or "being mentally ill." An example of this is hijacking your email address and sending out abusive emails to important people in your circle from your email address.
- **Stalking:** The narcissist may track your whereabouts, text or call continuously under the guise of co-parenting, but really they are trying to glean damaging information from you or set up a way to make themselves look better in the eyes of a third party, such as the courts. I have a client who gets continuous texts through an app where the court system can monitor interactions between

co-parents, in which her narcissist ex says things like "You know our son needs to be at a therapy session and you refuse to take him," so that the court might view her in a negative light . . . even though there isn't a therapy session scheduled!

The narcissist may stalk you and then accuse *you* of being the one doing the stalking.

- **Threats:** The narcissist will try to control their victims through the use of threats, which can become reality, fast. Threats from a narcissist are not always idle.

- **Legal Abuse:** When a narcissist uses the judicial system to smear you by creating false reports of child abuse or neglect, harassing you, impoverishing you, depleting you of finances due to exorbitant attorney's fees, or otherwise exerting control over you, this is legal abuse. Many of my clients are dragged into family court, which is a playground for narcissists. They often act the role of a loving and caring parent who wants to have more access to their children. Frequently, the narcissist will portray themselves as the victim of a mentally unstable co-parent and ironically demand psychological evaluations be done on the healthy parent (a form of gaslighting). Abusers and their lawyers often accuse protective parents of perpetrating *parental alienation*, which is a term debunked by therapists, and historically, used by some to try to spin the narrative.

CO-PARENTING AND POSTSEPARATION ABUSE

I've often said in this book that the narcissist will hit their victim where it hurts, and one of the worst ways I have seen postseparation abuse administered is when the narcissist turns the victim's children against them. Never is this truer than in the heat of a smear campaign when the narcissist is out for blood against the people they are "co-parenting" with. I put that word in quotes here because the narcissist actually *counter*parents.

- **Counterparenting:** The narcissistic parent will sow chaos into the lives of their ex-partners and children whenever they can. Many abusers don't mind hurting their children if they can harm their ex-partners in the process. They will complicate the transitions or exchange of possessions from one parent to the other, all while blaming the healthy parent in front of their children. They may even sabotage the children's efforts, such as by blocking their abilities to complete tasks, and then blame their healthy parent. Counterparenting also includes making phone calls and visitations as tense as possible. An example of this might be forcing a sick or injured child to FaceTime them or playing the victim if this does not occur.

- **Child Abuse/Neglect:** The narcissist may drive at dangerously high speeds with their child in the car; fail to protect the child adequately from getting sick, bug bites, diaper rash, or sunburn; allow the child to watch TV all day during their parenting time; or feed them exclusively junk food or even things that they know the child is allergic to. They love to block a mother from breastfeeding. If you try to tell them that the child has a food allergy, you can almost guarantee they will use that information against you and the child by feeding the child that food and blaming you for the medical fallout. They will try to groom a child to be a minion of theirs. Horrifically, they may even sexually abuse their children as a way to get back at their partner.

There is no worse version of postseparation abuse than when you have to navigate family court with a narcissist. There are more politics involved in the family court system because it works in a vacuum. There is no jury. You cannot speak of what happens there, publicly. There is no oversight, and many children are becoming traumatized by these horrifying practices. The narcissist will make up lies to damage your reputation in front of the very people who will be making custody decisions for you. In many cases, this leads to human trafficking. Let me explain.

While family courts are supposed to protect children, sometimes they do the exact opposite. Fortunately, there are some brave souls who are doing such important work in unveiling the corrupt family court system. One such person is Tina Swithin, founder of One Mom's Battle; her work in exposing "reunification camps," which are basically cults to reprogram children to do what the courts want them to do, blew the covers off the unlikely sources: These "camps" are often fueled by donations and monies given to corrupt judges via political campaigns or other efforts whereby the judges receive kickbacks from dirty attorneys or child custody evaluators or law guardians so that the judge does what they want the judge to do.[1]

On October 20, 2022, Maya (fifteen) and Sebastian (eleven) Laing were violently taken from their home after Judge Rebecca Connelly granted full custody to their mother and alleged abuser. The ruling called for Lynn Steinberg's "reunification camp" in Los Angeles, California, to hold Maya and Sebastian for days. They have subsequently been returned to their safe parent, but we are seeing stories like this all over the country.[2]

Others in the family court system have been under heavy scrutiny for taking bribes to be biased in custody cases.

My clients tell me of horrifying stories, with one woman having her children given to their abusive father, only to be abused by him and returned to their mother, with an apology from the court. Children literally being ripped from their safe family for money is human trafficking. Period. While this may sound far-fetched to some people (and others will be nodding their head), I spend most of my days helping my clients deal with a judicial system that doesn't get it, doesn't care, or both. We need to do more work here than anywhere.

YOU ARE NOT ALONE

Domestic violence has been visible throughout history and shows up in a variety of ways, from emotional abuse to acid attacks. In many cultures and time periods, women have had no rights and were instead possessions to be used for a dowry or to compensate the bride's family for the loss of her labor against her reproductive potential.

According to early Roman law, a man could beat, divorce, or murder his wife for any offenses committed by her that were seen to besmirch his honor or threaten his property rights. There were no rules against rape or any other crimes committed against a woman.

In the fifteenth century, the Catholic Church's endorsement of "The Rules of Marriage" perpetuated that a husband could stand as judge of his wife and was to beat her with a stick upon her commission of an offense. According to the "Rules," beating showed a concern for the wife's soul and well-being. The common law in England gave a man the right to beat his wife, in the interest of maintaining family discipline. In fact, the phrase "rule of thumb" originates in English common law, which allowed a husband to beat his wife as long as he used a stick that was no thicker than his thumb. Women were not the only ones subject to domestic abuse and public shaming. In eighteenth-century France, if it became public that a woman had beaten her husband, then he was forced to wear an outlandish costume and ride around the village backward on a donkey.

In the United States, it wasn't until the 1870s that the first laws banning a man's right to beat his family were passed. The laws were only moderately enforced until the second-wave feminist movement of the 1960s and '70s started bringing domestic violence to the attention of the media. By the 1980s, most states had adopted legislation regarding domestic violence. The Violence Against Women Act (VAWA), signed into law in 1994, provided $1.6 billion toward the investigation and prosecution of violent crimes against women; imposed automatic and mandatory restitution on those convicted; and allowed civil redress when prosecutors chose to not prosecute cases, but in 2021, 172 Republicans voted to oppose the renewal of the act, with many hell-bent on turning back the clock on women's rights, which of course does nothing to help the victims of narcissistic abuse. The United States is not the only country in which such travesties are happening. In Colombia, as well as Pakistan, India, Nepal, Bangladesh, and Uganda, women are still subjected to acid attacks, in which acid or another corrosive substance is thrown on a victim with the intent to maim, disfigure, torture, or even kill them. This extreme form of abuse demonstrates how threatened these women's abusers are by their beauty and independence.

To understand how our own society handles (or mishandles) narcissistic abuse, toxic masculinity, misogyny, and systemic patriarchy, we need to understand some of the numbers. It is indicated in the VAWA that domestic violence is the leading cause of injury to women in the United States. According to information released by the FBI about crime in the US, 89 percent of female murder victims were murdered by men. In 32 percent of these murders, the prime suspect was their husband or boyfriend. What's more, in 18.9 percent of reported rapes, a family member was the suspect. The FBI also estimated that one woman in the United States is beaten every eighteen seconds and that between 2,000 and 4,000 women will die each year from such abuse.[3]

Child abuse is fifteen times more likely to occur in families where domestic violence is present. Children who live in these environments are prone to trauma and to carrying on this abuse cycle with their own children.[4]

In the UK, as of 2020, there were some 2.3 million victims of domestic abuse a year ages sixteen to seventy-four (two-thirds of whom are women) and more than one in ten of all offenses recorded by the police are domestic abuse related, according to the government-provided fact sheet about 2021's Domestic Violence Act.[5]

While all these statistics are horrifying, people that are traumatized by narcissistic abuse also deal with invisible injuries, such as PTSD, and so I suspect the numbers of victims are far larger and the trauma for victims is exceedingly more pervasive than appears on the record.

SYSTEMIC FAILURES

Despite protections existing against domestic violence, narcissistic DV cases often fail to be prosecuted for a handful of reasons.

First, the judicial system is not savvy to what narcissistic abuse is. It is very hard to "catch" the narcissist in their devious behaviors because they are so slippery and sneaky. Mounting evidence against them can feel nearly impossible. Narcissists have been playing their games for a lifetime, so to outsmart them is a struggle, to say the least. It is more than likely that they have already gathered collateral to use against you *long before* you even realize who they are and what they are up to. They are skilled at creating a narrative that favors them in the court system and know exactly how to play up their "victimhood." Many of them make sure to educate themselves about attorney-client privilege and how to do consults with a bunch of attorneys—which makes those attorneys inaccessible to you.

Additionally, members of the judicial system may simply not care because they themselves are narcissists. When we talk about prosecutorial failures as they relate to narcissistic abuse, we have to talk about the ways in which our society looks at its hierarchical structures, especially as they relate to law enforcement. I cannot tell you how many clients have spoken to me about how the police mistreated them when they reported an abusive situation. They were made to feel stupid, overly emotional, or the reporting officer could even liken the victim to being "like my wife." As reported in *The Atlantic* in September 2014, research suggests that family violence is two to four times higher in the law enforcement community than in the general population.[6] We also see this within the military: the Department of Defense recorded forty-two thousand cases of domestic violence across all branches of the armed forces from 2015 to 2019.[7]

The most common response to domestic violence by the police and the courts is a restraining, or protective, order—a document that identifies the perpetrator as a potential threat to one victim (not to society in general) and instructs the abuser to have no physical or verbal contact with the victim. Although the information is inconclusive, 11 to 25 percent of women had an active restraining order against their abuser at the time of their murder. While there is some evidence of long-term benefit to a restraining order, initially there is a 21 percent chance of an escalation in violent behavior after an order of protection is issued.[8]

What we do know conclusively about restraining orders is that they can't guarantee safety as much as putting the perpetrator in jail does, but fewer than 2 percent of abusers ever receive any jail time. I am not saying that you shouldn't try to protect yourself with a restraining order but I am highlighting that the system has a long way to go to properly safeguard women and children. A 2012 report by the American Judges Association states that "Batterers have been able to convince authorities that the victim is unfit or undeserving of sole custody in approximately 70% of challenged cases."[9]

Many of my clients report providing piles of proof of domestic violence to the courts, which go on to ignore them in lieu of giving full parental custody to their abusers.

Beyond the courts, we have to look to society as a whole. Toxic masculinity hurts *everyone, including men.* Rigid traditional gender stereotypes prevent male victims of sexual assault from coming forward. Although 1 in 7 men have experienced physical violence, whether from a male or a female partner, the patriarchy shames men who are in domestically abusive situations away from seeking help. The perpetrator and the victim are both a symptom of the larger problem, patriarchy and gender inequality.

What's more, Child Protective Services (CPS) often fails victims of narcissistic abuse who are protective parents. They may blame the safe parent for staying with the abusive parent, when trying to get away would actually put everyone involved in more danger. Even if an abused woman decides to leave her partner, it may result in her becoming homeless, which puts her at risk of losing her kids.

So much work needs to be done to protect the narcissist's greatest source of exploitation—*their own children!* I cannot tell you how many victims of narcissistic abuse tell me that they are trying to get help getting away from an abuser, only to be revictimized by their own attorney and the entire judicial system. The judicial system is like a "mutual admiration society" for narcissists. From the police to the custody evaluators, these people can be far more toxic than you could ever imagine, and your entire life depends on their ability to not only *see* what you are trying to detail but to actually care!

EMOTIONAL AND PHYSICAL VIOLENCE

What was once a term for physical abuse, "domestic violence" has now expanded to include coercive control, intimidation, duress, and threats.

Consider this: Methods of mental and psychological torture the military is on record for having used include subjection to deafening noise; sleep disruption; sleep deprivation to the point of hallucination; deprivation of food, drink, and medical care; sexual humiliation; subjection to extreme heat or cold; and confinement. In addition to brutalizing detainees, there were threats to the family of detainees, such as threats to physically harm their children and threats to sexually abuse or to cut the throats of detainees' mothers.[10]

I highlight this here because it is so important for people to understand that **if the military, itself, considers these to be effective tactics to coerce and control detainees into doing what the military needs them to do, then why wouldn't we believe victims of narcissistic abuse are enduring some of these same tortures behind the scenes, in their own homes?** Domestic violence can be torture of the most insidious kind. Psychological abuse can leave someone feeling fearful, helpless, and powerless without anyone ever lifting a finger against them. Many of my clients who are physically abused express that the trauma of the emotional abuse they experienced is *far* worse.

According to the Centers for Disease Control and Prevention (CDC), 1 in 4 women has experienced violence from an intimate partner.[11]

A survivor of domestic violence and abuse does not need to experience physical abuse to be abused, but many do. What's more, dealing with physical abuse not only hurts your body but it also hurts you mentally. There are many types of physical abuse beyond "just" hitting. Some examples are:

- Hairpulling
- Slapping
- Burning
- Shoving
- Pinching
- Biting
- Twisting limbs
- Spitting

- Punching
- Kicking
- Making someone uncomfortable on purpose (e.g., taking their blanket or opening a window to make them cold)
- Physical restraint
- Confinement or involuntary isolation
- Rape and other forms of sexual abuse
- Incest
- Strangling

STRANGULATION

While this is a difficult matter to discuss, strangulation is an important element of physical domestic abuse to highlight here. This is because when an abuse victim is strangled, it greatly increases the risk of their becoming the victim of a homicide.

People often confuse choking with strangulation, so to clear up the confusion: choking is when an object blocks your airway, whereas strangulation is the presence of an outside force exerting enough pressure to block the movement of oxygen through your airway and to your brain. What's more, strangulation is often used in domestic abuse situations to control another person. It is one of the most lethal forms of domestic violence, because it has the potential to render the victim unconscious within seconds, dead within minutes. Most people who have been strangled by a domestic partner tend to downplay the act as "not serious"—in many cases, it is bad enough to set off alarms in the victim's mind, but not bad enough for them to do much about it—and *this is precisely what makes it so dangerous.* The narcissist will often "walk the line" and artfully fall under the radar by doing things to people that are slightly less physical than a direct hit.

Strangulation is one of the biggest safety issues victims of abuse face and should therefore be treated as not just a red flag, but as a bouquet of red flags. In fact, nonfatal strangulation is a significant predictor of future violence, and people who were strangled by their partner are at a risk six to ten times greater than average of being murdered by them.[12] Do not minimize the act! Press charges instead, and *do not* feel bad about reporting the incident. I cannot stress this enough. Strangulation is not only a gateway to further violence, but it can all too easily be overlooked. Many of my clients share horror stories of being strangled, even on their wedding night.

In August 2021, twenty-two-year-old Gabrielle Venora Petito was killed by her fiancé, Brian Laundrie, while they were traveling together on a cross-country road trip. The trip was planned to last for four months and began on July 2, 2021, but Petito disappeared in late August. Before she disappeared, many of the hallmarks of a domestic violence case reared their ugly head. A distraught Petito spoke to law enforcement in Moab, Utah, a few days before her death; the police report states that Petito hit Laundrie, likely reactive violence, but no arrests were made. After Laundrie strangled her, he showed true disregard of her personhood, abandoning her body to the Utah desert and returning to his home in Florida to die by suicide. Her body would not be found until three to four weeks after her estimated time of death.[13]

Rachel Louise Snyder points out in her book *No Visible Bruises: What We Don't Know About Domestic Violence Can Kill Us* that 60 percent of domestic violence victims are strangled over the course of an abusive relationship, and the overwhelming majority of stranglers (99 percent) are men. Those victims who lose consciousness are at the highest risk of dying twenty-four to forty-eight hours after the incident due to blood clots, stroke, or aspiration. Studies also now clearly show that a victim who is strangled once is a whopping 700 percent more likely to be seriously assaulted again and 800 percent more likely to become a victim of a homicide by their partner.[14]

Injuries from strangulation are often internal. Even in fatal cases, there are often no external signs of assault. While 50 percent of victims have visible injuries, only 15 percent can usually be photographed.[15] In emergency rooms across the country, victims are *not* routinely screened for strangulation or traumatic brain injury, and because the victims tend to have poor recall of the incident and a ton of cognitive dissonance, diagnoses are rarely formalized.

This is why a forensic exam is necessary to illuminate the skin to show where and how a woman has been strangled. An abuser knows signs of strangulation are much less noticeable than blunt force trauma, and will use this method before they resort to any other weapons. The abuser also knows the terror inflicted through strangulation. According to the *Journal of Emergency Medicine*, 97 percent of victims are strangled with hands, 38 percent report losing consciousness, 35 percent are strangled alongside sexual assault and abuse, and 70 percent believed they were going to die.[16] If a person has their hands around your neck, they're telling you they have the power to kill you.

In Alabama, the charge of domestic violence by strangulation or suffocation is a Class B felony, which means that, if convicted, the defendant faces a prison sentence of two to twenty years and a monetary fine of up to $30,000.[17] Sometimes, however, strangulation is charged as only a misdemeanor, even though half of all domestic violence homicides had prior strangulation and forty-eight states classify strangulation as a felony.

The narcissistic abuser literally has control of the woman's last breath, and what do we know about narcissists? They thrive on controlling others. If the victim survives, the psychological effects are also devastating. The fact is that, for too many people, strangulation is the last warning before their abuser succeeds in killing them. It's important for police officers, district attorneys, nurses, and doctors to educate themselves on where strangulation exists on the continuum of domestic violence. Only with appropriate education, charging, and sentencing can we break this potentially lethal progression of violence.

HOW DOMESTIC VIOLENCE CENTERS FALL SHORT

There is much work still to be done in the realm of DV centers, and this isn't to say that there aren't certain benefits they provide, but when it comes to the vernacular that victims of narcissistic abuse and cult abuse need to hear to feel validated, they can fall far short.

There are 13,500 animal shelters and rescue groups in the US compared to 1,887 DV programs, of which only 70 percent offer emergency shelter services.[18] This indicates a system that does little to support victims of domestic violence and their children, all while the judicial system is collectively guilty of retraumatizing victims.

There are often very few places to which women who flee their abusers can go that ensure their family's safety. Single women with children are more likely to live in poverty under normal circumstances, but add the complications that domestic abuse may bring—including being locked out of the house, locked out of their bank accounts, and trauma—and the postseparation period is so scary that people will elect to stay with their abusers. Half of all homeless women and children in the United States are fleeing an abusive home, and even though DV shelters are a temporary option for many of them, there are things that the shelters can improve upon. What follows are four concrete items, based on my personal first- and secondhand experience as a survivor of narcissistic abuse and as a therapist to other survivors, that DV centers can do to improve the ways they provide shelter and assistance to those who need it most.

FOUR THINGS DOMESTIC VIOLENCE CENTERS CAN DO TO IMPROVE

The first thing that DV centers need to stop doing is accepting money from known abusers.

Many DV centers function as nonprofits that depend on the donations of the community to run. In doing so, they get much of their financial backing from leaders of their communities, and what else do we know about narcissists? *They may be pillars of the communities they live in.* We need to stop protecting abusers and begin to call them out. Developing different ways to get funding should become a priority.

The second thing that DV centers need to do is get heavily involved in developing curriculum that supports phraseologies and vernacular that validate the victims, not just of domestic violence in general, but of narcissistic abuse in particular. As Dr. Daniel Siegel wittily asserts, "You have to name it to tame it." The value in using the correct words to describe a narcissist's characteristics is worth its weight in gold.[19]

When I did my run across New York State in a wedding dress to raise awareness for narcissistic abuse, I wanted to donate the monies I raised to DV centers in the respective counties that I ran through. However, not a single one of those centers would agree to receive the money under the concept of treating "narcissistic abuse." They believed that the clinical term in some way gave abusers a "pass"!

I couldn't disagree more. Under the current system in DV centers, when a survivor of narcissistic abuse escapes and arrives at a shelter, they could potentially stay in a confused state as to what happened to them. That is, until they hear the exact tactics that the narcissist uses—such as gaslighting, coercive control, isolation, triangulation—and until they learn about the clinical personality disorder that is associated with these characteristics, they may not connect the dots. Instead, they'll blame themselves and then find themselves back in that nightmarish environment.

Each and every client that comes to me needs to hear about the narcissist's playbook. They need to learn the equal parts horrifying and liberating truth that this had *nothing to do with them* and everything to do with a pathologically disordered individual. In other words, you cannot be responsible for it in any way because the narcissist does this to all their victims.

I would liken how DV centers mishandle this to walking into a hospital and having the hospital tell you that you are "sick." You would want to know what actually ails you. Is there a diagnosis, something to treat?! While we cannot diagnose a person's abuser (yet), it is of the utmost importance that we arm them with the language to do so. They need a comprehensive understanding of what they have endured and what the prognosis is to be able to step into their power and escape.

The third thing that DV centers need to do is keep a database of abusers they can reference if there is more than one victim of the same abuser. To avoid privacy issues, the victims would of course have to sign off on this, but if the greater good is explained to them, there may be room for growth here. Serial abusers repeat their tactics over and over, and this would be a great way to keep more people safe. Hopefully, one day we can have a national registry for narcissistic abusers.

This has to happen, because many people who leave a narcissist find themselves in the family court system, and this data could help support victims' cases in a colossal way! When I went to the DV center for support after I extricated myself from my abuser, they already knew that his ex-wife had used their services. I could have used this information to show the court the pattern of abuse that he had perpetrated against others over the years.

The fourth thing DV centers need to do is develop protocols for when one of their board members is abused. The board members of domestic violence centers are not always savvy to the words that we use in the clinical community to support DV victims. Most often, board members are random folks from the community, and many have not ever worked with this population before. They need to be trained to support all victims of narcissistic domestic abuse, including their fellow board members, in the same way that curriculum needs to be developed for the staff that trains them to support the victims that enter their programs.

SEEKING ASSISTANCE FROM ALTERNATIVES

I do not believe that domestic violence centers will help in understanding or escaping narcissistic abuse unless they can tell you that they have a specialist trained in handling narcissistic abuse on staff. If your local DV center does not have a specialist on staff and you are in need of help extricating yourself from a narcissist, your best course of action is to find a narcissist-savvy therapist. If money is tight, ask them about their sliding scale fee. I will never let a victim go without services because of money, and I am sure many of my cohorts feel the same way.

It is important to seek out such a specialist because you need the support of people who have gone through this, and many licensed therapists specializing in treating patients who've endured narcissistic abuse have also survived it themselves. It is almost an underground movement, a whisper network of therapists that are supporting this vulnerable population, and they will explain to you better than anyone else can how to navigate it and heal.

THERAPY TIP: NAME IT TO TAME IT[20]

To gently interrupt responses to triggers, you initiate "Name It to Tame It" after you notice your body's first response. It should look like this:

- You notice your body is telling you that you are feeling angry, afraid, or sad regarding a specific issue. You take in a deep breath.
- You recognize that you are getting upset, and without shaming yourself, you slowly exhale.
- You honestly name what happened to you and what you are feeling: anger or fear. You take in a slow breath.
- You notice your body slowly calming itself. You exhale again.
- You keep naming and breathing until you feel your body regulating.

Naming the emotions creates a kind of healthy distance between you and the reaction. You recognize the importance of experiencing the emotion, but you are not controlled by it.

Part III

Breaking Free

No matter where you are in your journey, whether you are just beginning to be able to acknowledge your trauma or if you have gotten out of the relationship but still need to level up, this part of the book is meant to help you heal. From getting the hell out to healing tips, these chapters are my gift to you. You can read them in order or you can skip to Chapter 17 to find practical healing exercises.

Chapter 16

"Run Like Hell!"— Creating an Exit Strategy

I remember what it felt like when I first fled my abusive relationship. There was the pain and confusion of not just that loss, but the loss of so many other relationships. Even so, I would not change a single thing. I became stronger with each passing day. My friendships grew truer. The trust I developed within myself is unbreakable, and I began to lean into becoming the most empowered version of myself.

───❧───

By now, you know that, by and large, narcissists will not change and do not want to change. Therefore, your main recourse is to leave. Creating an exit strategy may be tricky, though. You may want to scream at them and let them know what you have discovered, but I don't recommend this. It is far better to quietly gather your evidence of their abuse and your belongings, make plans with trusted friends and family, and find a place to stay while you get your life back together.

I won't sugarcoat it. This can be a long, scary, and arduous process, but though it is going to take a long time to heal, it is so worth it! You will become a more intuitive person who is stronger than you ever thought you could be. You will discover who is a true friend versus who is a toxic person who may have burdened you mentally for years. You will become less judgmental of others and more rooted in your empathetic side. This is your rebirth; you are finally on the path to a healthier version of yourself. There are stages to getting away that include the following.

- **Precontemplation Stage:** where there does not seem to be a problem
- **The False Optimism Stage:** where you see red flags, but convince yourself that everything is going to be fine
- **The Contemplation Stage:** where you see red flags and are not sure what to do
- **The Preparation Stage:** where you start to gather information and consider options
- **The Action Stage:** where you start to leave, divorce, and go no contact

Many people get hoovered back in, so it is imperative to maintain your boundaries and distance!

OKAY, SO WHAT NOW?!

After you recognize that you've been through the phases of narcissistic abuse, you may want to get justice. There are ways to do so if you play your cards right. Unfortunately, though, invariably and ironically, the courts are often the biggest barriers to justice, so let's get you as insulated as possible with resources, especially against potential abuses of the legal system.

Get a narcissist-savvy therapist. The first and foremost thing you should do after getting away from the narcissist is to seek counseling. It cannot be overstated enough that counseling after this type of abuse is paramount to healing, but it can also be helpful to you in any court cases you may now face.

While we will get into the therapeutic value of talking to a psychologist or mental health counselor more in the next chapter, you must lay the groundwork regarding the damage that has been done to your psyche with a licensed professional in the mental health field. This is especially true if you've developed trauma as a result of your abuse. It is the only diagnosis with liability, meaning that something or someone caused it.

In addition to having a written record of your abuse, it is superimportant to open up about your emotions in the safe space of a therapist's office. That way, you avoid internalizing this toxicity, and you're more emotionally composed in court! After you deal with a narcissist, it's only natural to feel a range of negative emotions, such as frustration and sadness, and to experience trauma or triggers, both known and unknown. To be able to show up to a trial hearing as your most cool and collected self, speak with a mental health professional first. You'll not only get some relief, but you'll also be able to strategize about how you'll describe your experiences to the court if necessary.

Anyone who's faced narcissistic abuse has likely experienced isolation, but a trained counselor can help you open up about your circumstances. This way, you can feel heard, get it out of your system, and process it all, moving forward. A mental health professional can also point out signs of abuse you might have missed, so that you can include them in your documentation. They can help you put words to the craziness that you have experienced and help you learn to cope through various, proven therapy practices and perspectives that heal your mind, body, and soul.

Could you try to do this alone or with a garden-variety psychotherapist? Sure. But if you try to do it alone or without the support of a psychotherapist who specializes in narcissistic abuse, you not only run the risk of meeting another narcissist, but if a therapist does not understand what this is, they may push you back into the arms of a monster, or it could take years longer to recover. Consider finding the right therapist your first and best line of defense.

You can search for therapists who specialize in narcissistic abuse at
PsychologyToday.com, or you might look for a therapist who specializes in treating survivors of domestic violence. Interview them and ask
them about their own experience with narcissists. You might also visit
TellATherapist.org to be put in touch with a narcissist-savvy clinician or
attorney in your area. Look for a therapist who understands what gaslighting is and can readily describe some of the terms found in this book.
If they cannot, you could have serious problems. In short, find a therapist who "gets it."

I've provided some links in the Resources section (pages 275–277) on
how to find a therapist. Here are some questions you can ask a therapist to
determine whether they are a good fit for you.

- Do you have experience with narcissistic personality disorder
  (NPD) or treating victims of narcissists?
- Do you have experience working with domestic violence survivors?
- What methods of therapy do you use?
- Do you take insurance? Do you have a sliding scale?

If you'd like to take a smaller step before reaching out to a therapist
over the phone or online, these final chapters, on having an exit strategy
and on healing, should be useful.

DEALING WITH LEGAL ABUSE

If you are dealing with a particularly litigious abuser, it is important
to prepare for any dealings with the judicial system. Here are some suggestions:

Create a paper trail of the narcissist's abuse. Prepare to show the
courts that you took action ASAP to make sure you and your children
(if you have them) are safe and to prevent your abuser from creating a
smear campaign. Document every infraction and record every move you
make. Do not use the phone to communicate with the narcissist unless
you record your conversations, as they can expose themselves in these

conversations. Use text messages or emails to engage with them, so that everything is recorded and readily accessible. In short, pretend you are making a *Dateline*-esque documentary about your story. Imagine that all interactions are being viewed by a judge and jury and chronicle them accordingly. The narcissist is going to do this against you, so try to get ahead of them at every stage of the game.

Additionally, contact a domestic violence advocate (see Resources, pages 275–277, for info on how to find one) and have them document what you have experienced. You might want to get a restraining order if your abuser is doing what they normally do: harassing and stalking you after the relationship ends. A restraining order is designed to keep your abuser from contacting you. It is an especially good idea if you know or suspect they have a firearm, but keep in mind, it is far better to avoid family court if at all possible. If you can get into a civil court or a criminal court, you will get in front of a jury and not a potentially corrupt judge. In other words, if you already have any agreements in place, look to go for a breach of contract and stay away from family court, if possible. You can even file reports with the police that the narcissist never has to learn about. To do this, go to a police station when the narcissist does things to harass you, and have the police document their behaviors so that you can present that information later as needed. They do not have to file charges or even alert your abuser, but it goes a long way to make these efforts to protect yourself and your children.

Encourage others to vouch for you and your integrity. Request "character reference letters"—written statements from the people who are closest to you, such as friends, relatives, or coworkers. Prioritize people who have known you for a long time, ideally longer than the abuser has been in your life, and who have lots of background knowledge about you— bonus points if they have strong credentials or an impressive background themselves. Ask these people to expand on your strong morals and values, especially if you have no arrest record or substance abuse history. If you end up in court, this will help enhance your reputation and explain how reasonable you are. Many do not end up in court with a narcissist, but so many people are not as fortunate.

Take a voluntary drug test. I cannot tell you how many narcissists project their substance abuse onto their victims. They will act as though they have endured years of abuse at the hands of you, an alcoholic or drug-addicted spouse, while you are the one who has been victimized by their alcoholism or drug addiction.

Get witnesses to your abuse to share what they saw. Reach out to anyone you know who saw what happened to you, such as teachers, family members, friends, or neighbors who were present anytime you had a dispute with the narcissist and/or anytime the narcissist mistreated you. Make sure that what they saw aligns with the facts as well as with your testimony or personal account.

If the narcissist baited you into reacting negatively or violently to them in a public place and people saw it, get them to share what they saw, in written or recorded form, if they are willing. Request write a "witness statement" that outlines what they experienced and sign it to confirm that it's true. Witness statements can include what a person saw, heard, or felt when they were around the narcissist. Ask them to make it robust and then check it to make sure it is accurate. If it's notarized, even better! If the witnesses do not even know you that well, that is perfectly fine! They have no loyalty to you and therefore might be considered an even better witness than one who is partial to you and your cause.

Start interviewing attorneys and get the sharkiest. If you think it's too early to hire a lawyer, remember that many narcissists use family court as their own personal playground during the falling-out phase of a relationship. You will likely need one, and you will want one who is not only narcissist-savvy but has a good success rate.

If that set off some alarm bells for you, let me explain. You want an attorney who understands exactly what narcissism is. It is even better if they know how to "play the game" because these attorneys do not want to lose. They will be employing one-upmanship as well as, if not better than, your abuser does.

The attorney who hates to lose and employs rogue tactics to find loopholes and ways to play the system is generally better for your purposes than is the neurotypical attorney. A regular attorney or mediator will not be much help in a court battle against a narcissist because there is no negotiating with someone who truly has narcissistic personality disorder. Forget about mediation. This is a waste of time, money, and resources. This is war. The narcissist will play games and use tactics to exhaust your resources. A narcissist will risk everything they have to destroy you, even if it means their own self-destruction.

With all this in mind, ask people in your community who the "sharkiest" attorney is, then research the politics of your local family court. Find the most cutthroat lawyer who is "in bed" with the heavy hitters in your region. This is not a joke. Lawyer selection will change the trajectory of your life, especially if you have children. Many people lose custody to their abusers, so wisely invest in choosing the right lawyer. You have to understand the politics and learn who's who in your region. Your attorney needs to be close to the judges. Period. This might sound ridiculous. It is not. I assure you.

Gather your documentation. Once you've retained a lawyer, with your help, they'll put together their case of evidence against your abuser. A *subpoena* is an order that requires an individual to appear in court to share their account with the judge and to substantiate (verify) that a narcissist has abused you before and that you've handled yourself with grace and composure. A subpoena served to the right person can help substantiate your claims of abuse and help you protect yourself.

You can also use a subpoena for documents important to your case, such as proof that a narcissist was involved in a previous domestic abuse case, never paid child support, or has a history of violence. Many people also conduct forensic financial reports to corroborate their finances and the finances of their abuser for child support and alimony. They can also request forensic biological, psychological, and/or social reports that they can gather from a skilled professional to prove that your abuser has a disorder or that you do not.

This can be risky. Many of the psychiatrists and psychotherapists in the judicial system are not savvy to narcissistic abuse and may be heavily involved in the local politics of that family court system, as I mentioned earlier. In other words, they may be more inclined to support the clients of an attorney with whom they have worked well previously.

Do your research into how forensic psychologists in the family court report on domestic violence cases. Many have a reputation of siding with known abusers, so again, hiring a sharky, narcissistic attorney who's "in the know" and can game this corrupt system is in your best interest.

Learn the laws as they relate to DV and housing. If you are experiencing housing issues, financial issues, or are otherwise unable to pay your rent as a result of your abuser, you may be entitled to break your lease as a victim of DV. There are certain laws that protect victims in certain districts. Reach out to legislators in your area to see what housing options are available to you. See Resources, pages 275–277, for links.

Remain calm. You cannot succeed in court if you are not cool, calm, collected, and clinical in your presentation. Remaining reposed also checks another very important box in a court of law: Your lack of reactions could upset the narcissist to the extent that they reveal their true selves to the court. The calmer you behave, the more likely they are to become agitated and let their mask slip.

Since an abusive person thrives off power dynamics and stirring up negative feelings, don't give them the satisfaction. Discuss only the facts and objective details of the case. Leave your emotions at the door. You may want to throw up or feel that you are going to break out in hives, but this calm version of you will pay dividends later. When you remain mature as you address the way you've been mistreated, you'll expose the narcissist for who they truly are. As a consequence, they're likely to melt down in court and engage in melodrama, over-the-top stories, or histrionics, which will hopefully cause the judge to take your side.

Narcissists often need constant praise and attention, so if you, your attorney, or your witnesses critique them, a narcissist is unlikely to remain levelheaded. If a narcissist does make degrading comments or lose their temper in court, then the judge is likely to compare that to any documentation that suggests they are abusive. Some narcissists will even become reactive and fight with your lawyer, or text you from a burner phone to distract or unnerve you. This is all part of their game. Stay cool. This only indicates that they are nervous.

I'm not saying it's easy to remain calm in the courtroom. You are likely being revictimized by the narcissist's nasty attorneys and pummeled by the lies that they have been fed by your abuser, but breathe through it, and remember the truth. Remember that you are the victor—you have been ever since you got away from them—and you are on the road to safety.

In court, address only the judge or the court officer that is engaging with you. This choice helps you ignore any of the narcissist's intimidation tactics—and there will be many. They may even make hand signals, when nobody is looking, that they are going to shoot you in the head or cut your throat. The narcissist may have a habit of chuckling, glaring at you, clicking a pen, or making rude side remarks from their seat. Ignore them. When your attorney or the narcissist's lawyer asks you any questions, look toward the judge and answer in a neutral tone of voice. Make it clear that you're speaking to the court officers and the judge. Thank the judge when you can.

A narcissist might try to pull at your heartstrings and play the victim to make you pity them. They may cry fake tears and act in a variety of pathetic ways; they are great actors, but it can be hard to keep up with their lies. If you avoid any eye contact with them, you'll be able to think clearly.

Don't sign anything that compromises your voice or takes away your rights. Once the judge has made their decision, avoid any compromises that the abuser asks for. Remember that you cannot negotiate with narcissists—they will try to appeal to a "fair" deal and then go back on their word anyway. Any outcomes, such as the full custody you received or a divorce that you were granted, are court ordered and they need to respect them. Anytime they deviate from court orders, let the court know straightaway, even if it is busying, because you have to protect yourself from future judicial dealings.

Never sign a nondisclosure agreement! Beyond trying to get you to compromise on court-ordered decisions, the narcissist may try to get you to sign a nondisclosure agreement about your time together. If you do, you are only assured of one thing: that you have given your power and voice away. This is the kiss of death for many victims because the narcissist goes on to continue their abusive behaviors, leaving you with little recourse to help yourself, since you cannot speak your truth. Lawyers may try to get you to sign civil restraints. I do not recommend this, because you will similarly sign your voice away. Civil Restraints are like NDA's little brother and we need our voices if things are to change for future generations.

FURTHER DOS AND DON'TS OF LEAVING AN ABUSIVE RELATIONSHIP

You may want to scream, punch, kick, throw something, or get revenge once you've left a narcissistic relationship, and believe me, I get it. It is so maddening to deal with this and to do it alone, but it is important to lean on others so that you can outsmart the narcissist. There will be tons of things you *want* to do, but that does not mean you should do them.

Here are some things you will *want* to do, but that may not be advisable:

- *Tell the world what you have endured.* They might not even believe it, given how hard it is for you to believe.
- *Expect your abuser to receive justice.* The judicial system, for the most part, doesn't get it and doesn't care . . . yet.
- *Underestimate* the narcissist's ability to win you over
- *Believe* you need closure to move on. Make your own closure.
- *Listen* to flying monkeys trying to drag you back into the hell of the relationship
- *Empathize* with the narcissist

Meanwhile, here are some things that you may not want to do but will *need* to do:

- Find a safe space to go when you leave. Move to a new location if you have the resources. Many people report to me that a move to a new region was a huge step toward healing.

- Limit or go "no contact" with the narcissist (depending on whether you share children or not).
- Change your phone number and *all* online passwords. Block social media accounts.
- Get a security system for both the outside and inside of your home. Be able to prove where you are at all times. I had to do this, but it was worth the effort. It really helped me in court.
- Get a dashcam.
- Open a separate bank account unless you're going through a divorce. If so, refer to your state's laws about this matter first.
- Alter your appearance (e.g., change your hair color or style) if you fear that you are being targeted or followed.
- Ween yourself off the drug that was your narcissist.
- Begin to *detach*.
- Become forward-thinking and savvy. Anticipate all the ways the narcissist will fight back or retaliate, and preemptively counteract those moves to the best of your ability.
- Acclimate back into the real world. Unhand many of the fantastical thoughts that the narcissist methodically planted in your brain through gaslighting and manipulation tactics.
- Grieve, not only what you thought you had and all the versions of your abuser that you liked, but the social concept of the fairy tale you've been fed through the media and others.
- Prepare for the vindictive and vengeful version of your abuser to rear its ugly head, and prepare for it all as safely as possible, especially if *you* left *them*.
- Become independent emotionally, mentally, physically, and financially.
- Build up a support team that you can rely on and trust.
- Document the narcissist's behavior.
- Make statements of abuse (where applicable) to the police to record your account.
- Practice self-care.
- Get counseling.

TELL A THERAPIST'S HIERARCHY OF RESTORATION

Soul Restoration Pyramid

"Recovery from Narcissistic Abuse"

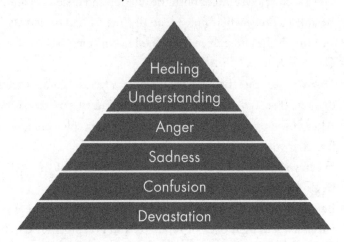

Similar to Maslow's Hierarchy of Needs, in which we seek increasingly elevated fulfillment in our lives, or like Elisabeth Kübler-Ross's framework for grief, you will go through certain phases after you are free from your abuser. I call these the *Phases of Instating Sovereignty:*

Devastation

Confusion

Sadness

Anger

Understanding

Healing

Devastation

This is a hard but not entirely unexpected phase of recovery; after all, you've just endured the Ultimate Betrayal—that it was all a *lie*! After the realization that the narcissist is nothing more than a charming mirage, the devastation can be tremendous; you will feel a level of betrayal that you may never have felt before. You may feel that you are broken emotionally, sexually, and physically, but you are not! You are experiencing a "leveling-up," though it sure as shit doesn't feel like it when you are going through it.

When we are children, we are taught that people are innately "good," and so it can feel scary after you leave the narcissist or are discarded by them, but when you accept that some people, deep down, are just as deviant as they present themselves on the surface, you are learning a painful but valuable truth.

Eventually, you will be able to put this truth to use, finding the people who are truly worth your time, love, and energy! Believe me when I tell you that they are out there and they are the most precious creatures. Look for the silver linings. The universe will bring you the safe people. The key is to have enough openness to welcome them in and an equal amount of savviness to keep the disordered people out.

Confusion

Being mirrored and gaslit for so long may make you think that you are the toxic one and that this devastation is all your fault. You will likely experience cognitive dissonance. Whenever you're made to believe one thing one day and then the entire conversation is denied the next, or you were swept off your feet in a shower of affection and attention, only to be ignored or abandoned the following day, the result is a purposeful, deep, and profound confusion about not just the relationship but about everything! Was it *all* a lie? Was the person you were with the wonderful and charismatic person, or are they the abusive, emotionally unavailable, and cold person they're presenting to you now? Is the truth what was discussed in detail over the last few years, or is it the denial of the conversations, promises, and agreements you've endured lately? You may begin to feel that you are going crazy, trying to piece together what is fact and what is fiction.

Sadness

You may feel anguished after you clear up the confusion, as if you are in free fall. You may experience depressive symptoms and may feel so supremely ashamed that you isolate yourself from others even further. Symptoms of depression may include difficulty concentrating, fatigue, irritability, feelings of guilt, worthlessness, loss of appetite, overeating, pain, and/or digestive problems. You may develop an inability to connect with others on a deep, intimate level, as well as self-doubt, low self-esteem, exhaustion, and a weakened immune system.

Anger

Once they move past their sadness, many survivors of narcissistic abuse are surprised to learn they feel a great deal of rage. The level of fury may vary, but many people have spent twenty to thirty years of their life wasting time on a con artist! Many are so devastated personally, professionally, and financially that they may need many years to climb out of the hole.

If you're going through anger, don't cheat yourself out of it or lean away from it as though it's an ugly emotion. I prefer that my clients experience anger and process it, so they can move on to practice love. So as not to internalize the pain you are feeling, it is actually healthy to feel and manage your anger. Go to a rage room or scream into a pillow, if you must, but try to express it and let it out. I find audio journaling is great for this.

Understanding

Most of your time and energy after getting away from a narcissist should be spent getting clarity about what you have gone through. This takes a long time, so be patient. Research it. Learn about it. Become confident in the truth, which will set you free. Learning about this personality disorder, and all the pain that it causes, will also make you realize that you are not alone, and the presence of others who know what you've been through will be extremely validating.

Healing and Self-Actualization

At the very beginning of this book, when we talked about safety, we discussed Maslow's hierarchy. Now we are going to talk about it again, but with a focus on the "self-actualization" part of the pyramid. This section of this chapter and the last chapter of the book are about how to meet your potential and heal, so if you don't feel ready for that or feel you are still too stuck in your abuse recovery, that is 100 percent okay! It may still add value to read through it, though, because it can be that subtle whisper to you that you are going to be all right. If you still think it is too hard, come back to these pages when you are ready.

As a humanist, Maslow believed that people have an innate tendency toward self-actualization. To achieve these ultimate goals, though, a number of more basic needs must first be met, such as the need for food, shelter, and clothing. After all, it's difficult to become self-actualized when you don't know where you'll get your next meal.

Even so, Maslow emphasized the importance of self-actualization, which is a process of growing. He termed the highest level of the pyramid as growth needs, and these needs don't stem from a lack of something, rather from a desire to grow as a person—to "meet your potential." At the very peak of the hierarchy pyramid are the self-actualization needs. According to Maslow's definition of self-actualization, "It may be loosely described as the full use and exploitation of talents, capabilities, potentialities, etc. Such people seem to be fulfilling themselves and to be doing the best that they are capable of doing. They are people who have developed or are developing to the full stature of which they can be capable."[1] Self-actualizing people are less concerned with the opinions of others. Instead, they are self-aware and are more interested in personal growth and fulfilling their potential. The goal is to become solid in your self-esteem and move through barriers with confidence. Everybody's version of self-actualization is different, but here are some things to put into practice:

- **Live an Authentic Life.** Being truly honest, especially with oneself, is a method of taking responsibility. This is the place of ultimate growth—a place that the narcissist will never visit!
- **Be Present.** Remain present in a selflessly vivid way, with full concentration on what you are currently experiencing. This means you are living your best life when you are highly engaged in the moment.

- **Be Aware of Your Choices.** When we learn to classify our choices as progressive or regressive, we can get into healthier patterns that only involve growth.
- **Get to Know Yourself.** Get to know who you are without the noise that may have been inputted over the years by parents, friends, abusive partners, or anyone else. Learn about your strengths and weaknesses without the pressure of what others think about you. Who are you, really? What are you passionate about? What inspires you? What do you enjoy? What makes you feel moved and joyful? Rather than consult society, your peers, or the establishment about how you should feel and think about something, get to know your internal self. Far more often than we realize, we download our opinions from authority, but it's in our opinions that we can identify our true selves.
- **Do Not Worry About What Others Think.** When you come out of an abusive relationship with a narcissist and have spent so much time being gaslit and lied to, you can have a hard time figuring out how to trust people and even yourself. However, if you do the work and buddy up to other survivors who have gone through it, it is my belief that you will have a better chance of reaching self-actualization than someone who has not gone through this. Why? Because you have seen something remarkable, endured the doubt and victim-blaming from your abuser and from society as a whole, and come out on the other side. Based on this, your ability to see bullshit and seek the truth is more refined. You will become far more attuned to what truth is and how to not be swayed from it in spite of what the masses may believe. What a gift! This may make you unpopular, but at this stage, you won't care!
- **Never Stop Growing.** People who are self-actualized never "retire" from the journey of growth. They are perpetually curious and always working toward their betterment and the betterment of others.
- **Notice Universal "God-Winks."** When you "stop and smell the roses" or take notice of the beauty and wonder in life, you are not

only being present in the moment and practicing gratitude; you are also fully aware of how small you are in the universe. You understand how trivial things are, and you unhand your ego. Taking notice of the universe's gifts and winks is a special treasure in our lives, and can bring us to a place where we become less ego-driven and more connected to the bigger picture.

- **Accept Your Shortcomings.** When you can identify the less pleasant parts of yourself and still love yourself entirely, you may come to value yourself even more than you did before. Nobody is perfect; we all have strengths and weaknesses. Understanding this duality of the good in you and the bad parts of you is a strong indication that you are reaching self-actualization.

Self-actualized people are reality- and problem-centered and can distinguish what is fake and dishonest from what is real and genuine. They enjoy being by themselves, and have deeper relationships with a few people, instead of more shallow relations with many people. They tend to be *autonomous*, and have a sense of what is true beyond their culture, are highly resistant to culturalization, and thus enjoy being themselves without worrying about fitting in. They are spontaneous, nonconforming, and have humility. They are creative, fresh, and original in their ideas and moved by forces larger than themselves.

—∞∞—

Even though this chapter provides some good tips to building your exit strategy, it doesn't mean that your story and the difficulty you've experienced in getting away from your abuser are not honored or appreciated. It can be difficult to cope with the emotions and feelings of the letdown that comes with realizing your fairy-tale ending isn't coming with this person, but it is possible to live a far better life after ridding yourself of the narcissist than you could ever imagine.

THERAPY TIP: ADDITIONAL HELP FOR
YOUR EXIT

Here are some additional tips for handling your exit well:
HIDE MONEY! This is so important. Do this straightaway.
Recognize that it's not your fault. IT'S NOT YOU! The best and worst parts of this relationship are the same: It had nothing to do with you. This truth is equal parts liberating and horrifying. It is liberating because the narcissist never even saw you (so it is not your fault) and horrifying for the exact same reason.
Recognize that they will do the exact same thing to their next supply. They will, 100 percent, continue in their behaviors. Hard stop, but this is the sad truth for the next supply and it can be horrifying to watch, but forget about what you see on social media, how they seem to have circled back around to Prince Charming in all the pictures they post with their new supply. Get off social media if you have to. In the wise words of Public Enemy, "Don't believe the hype. It's a sequel."
Distract yourself. When you return to doing things that make you happy, such as spending time with friends or taking time for yourself, you'll realize that you're better off without the abusive relationship. This, in turn, will make it easier to move on to other things. Get back to the person you were before this, or discover the next best version of yourself. Look for things that make you laugh and feel free.
Stay connected to people who get it. Your support system should be strong and filled with your fellow survivors of narcissistic abuse—people who have experienced this and know where you're coming from.
Recognize your own strengths. We all have strengths. Lean into yours and think daily about what they are. You will want to change your thought patterns to remember this, which might be

easier said than done. A person who has experienced trauma may even develop obsessive-compulsive disorder and have very rigid ways of thinking, which are hard to shift away from. If you were in a relationship with a narcissist, you may have developed some tunnel vision or severe thought patterns. You need to shift away from those pathways and get into different ways of thinking.

Think about when you were a kid and you went sledding on the neighborhood's most popular sleighing hill. Your sled would automatically enter the lanes in the snow that were made by the people who had sled before you. That is, in many ways, how our thought patterns develop. They can become so ingrained in your neural networks, especially if you have an intense, traumatic experience to really drive them down deep. You need some clean and untouched snow to sled on. Open your mind and think differently. Push yourself toward self-love and shift away from your old way of thinking. The narcissist may have made their own track, forcing you to think negatively about yourself, but make your own way forward. Begin to think positively about yourself instead.

Don't stoop to their level. This may be tempting, but a narcissist is the petulant child who is desperate for you to react in the ways that you have done historically. Don't take the bait. Resist the urge to defend yourself if your narcissist reaches out to you or bad-mouths you in public. Recognize that this behavior has nothing to do with you and everything to do with them. Remain calm, take their insults in stride, and choose not to accept them.

Knowing how to emotionally detach from a narcissist can be highly useful when you're leaving an abusive relationship with one. Leaving may not be easy, but cutting off emotional ties and recognizing that you are not to blame for their behavior are important steps in the process.

Chapter 17

Healing

After I got away from my abusive ex, I came up with this idea that I was going to run across the entire state of New York in a wedding dress to raise awareness for narcissistic abuse, and that's just what I did! I was free, I was determined, and I was not backing down. My story and the stories of the millions of victims that suffer in silence needed to be told. The power that I felt in speaking the truth was scary, but it was so worth it. You are worth it. We are worth it! Every step I took in my white sneakers across those 285 miles was a step into my power, my healing, and my freedom. I felt as if every one of the silent victims was running with me across the Empire State.

Similarly, you should feel not just me alongside you on this journey but all the other victims who have endured something eerily similar to what you have survived. You will prevail, and you are never alone in this journey.

If you have gotten away from a narcissist, you are primed for self-actualization. You have seen the darkest parts of humanity. Now, the only way out is up! You have been given the gift of understanding, and can take this intel and turn that pain into power. You can begin to live

*a life where you can focus on yourself and become the best version
of you! Your next chapter is the one where you are free to be whatever you want. People are going to think what they want about you
anyway, so why not take this opportunity to turn this ship around and
be the absolute truest version of yourself? I know I work toward this
every day, and it has been the most liberating experience of my life.*

N o matter where you are in your journey, I'd like you to take a moment
to acknowledge all the hard work you've done to reach this point.
Recognizing that we've been victims of narcissists can be tough, extracting ourselves, even more so. This chapter will serve as the light to guide
you through the healing process. During the healing process, which can
seem like it takes forever, these lessons can help anyone who is in recovery feel proactive. Being victimized by a narcissist feels like death by a
thousand cuts, but this chapter can stop the bleeding and get you not only
whole again but living the life that you deserve! In this chapter, there will
be something for everyone in almost every stage of the healing process,
though it mostly focuses on dealing with the postseparation experience,
which is the most abusive for many victims.

I will start by offering up some tangible, pragmatic, and empirical
ways to soothe, repair, and rehabilitate the parts of you that are in pain
and need mending, including developing your support network. I will then
talk about ways to level up and work toward meeting your potential and
making your dreams come true.

No matter where you are in your journey, I advise against reading this
chapter all at once, which would likely feel like drinking from a fire hose.
Instead, I encourage you to take your time. Maybe hop around to the sections that resonate with you or come back to the weightier exercises after
giving yourself a few weeks to process what you've already learned about
yourself.

I recommend you buy a journal to write in or create a journal on your computer; some of the exercises ask you to take notes and give you things to contemplate, and having a dedicated journal can be a great safe space for you to record your feelings and responses.

Paramount to your healing is the creation of distance between yourself and your narcissistic abuser. You will find that your perspective becomes clearer with every passing day that you are away from them. Second to that distance is becoming educated on what sort of relationship you were in. About 80 percent of your early days of recovery will be spent learning about and processing what you have undergone. It is a hard thing to do, so we dedicate a good amount of time to becoming experts on our own experiences.

Don't feel bad about this. It gets less and less difficult over time, but the healing process does take time. I tell my clients it can take two to four years of recovery. I know this sounds like a lot, but the first six months generally are the most intense—and likely will be the worst, in all honesty. It will all improve, albeit slowly. Educating ourselves on what narcissism is and how it works is the most valuable way we as survivors can spend our time. If you neglect to do this, you may find yourself repeating the same patterns again with another abuser, so *do the work*! Understanding the narcissist's playbook will help take the burden off you and release you from any self-blame you may be experiencing. Once you have done this work, you can truly begin to heal!

Some of the healing practices in this chapter are clinical, while others may feel more "life-coachy," but they are all extremely valuable and will help you have the best possible outcomes in your healing process. You have more than likely experienced trauma, so the tools and resources provided here can help you deprogram from unhealthy behaviors and thought processes, and instead develop more positive neural pathways to help you recover.

Many of us stayed with our abuser for so long because we believed the lies they told us. Many of us were too confused to make sense of what was even happening to us. There are a variety of reasons why we endured narcissistic abuse for as long as we did, and that's okay! We all had our reasons. As a first step on this healing journey, let's take a quick look at why many stay.

- Fear of the unknown
- False hopes
- Thinking they're "too old" to be alone and/or start anew
- To keep the house
- To share the housework and responsibilities
- Guilt
- For the kids
- Fear of being alone
- For the money/financial reasons
- Fear of others' reactions
- Nostalgia for the good old days
- Sex
- Having the same friends
- Blackmail, emotional or financial
- To avoid feelings of failure
- Hopefulness that promises will be kept
- Thinking, "Maybe [their abuser] will change"
- Cultural or religious reasons

Keeping this list of reasons in mind should help you validate for yourself that you are not alone. Many people have struggled to leave abusive relationships, and unfortunately, you won't be the last.

Now that we know why many victims stay with their abusers, let's identify some key things you need to do to create your ideal healing environment. First is understanding your *why*.

CORE WOUNDS

Core wounds are often traumas from childhood, such as not feeling good enough or feeling stupid. If you are able to peel back the onion layers and find your core wound, you are in a much better place. For me, it was the abandonment by my father at the age of nine and bullying by schoolmates from an early age. When I discovered that that little girl felt "not good enough" or "unworthy" her entire life, I understood what void I was trying to fill by choosing partners that were not emotionally available or engaging in unhealthy habits and the work I needed to do to feel worthy and good enough. I started to work with a therapist, and developed mantras and a strong support system that reminded me daily of my value and why my father had done the best he could. I journaled to process it all and forgive the people around me that had hurt me at a young age. I could, then, stop trying to fix my pain and feelings of shame. This work is extremely hard and extremely important but is best done with a trained professional. When I was in court one day with my abuser, I could feel my father standing next to me lean down and whisper in my ear, "I never left you" and this felt very healing for me—the idea that he was always with me, in spirit. One of the other tricks that helped me was a little gift given to me by my dear friend and soul sister, Nicole. She offered me the "RAIN" method of meditation, whereby you Recognize, Allow, Investigate, and Nurture. I'll share that here with you.

When you are feeling triggered, try this:

- **Recognize** what you are feeling. Are you sad? Mad?
- **Allow** yourself to feel it.
- **Investigate** what you are feeling and why. What is the origin?
- **Nurture** by telling yourself, "It's okay, sweetheart," or you might just say to yourself, "I love you" or "It's okay, I'm here. I'm not leaving."

FIND YOUR PEOPLE

Research has shown that there are tremendous benefits to having a network of supportive relationships. Those with robust social support networks have better health, longer lives, and overall greater well-being. Friends and loved ones can make you more resilient in times of stress, setback, or loss; can help prevent you from going back to bad habits; and can make the good times even better. Stable, healthy friendships are crucial for our well-being and longevity. People who have friends and close confidants are more satisfied with their lives and less likely to suffer from depression.[1] Additionally, supportive relationships can bolster you emotionally when you're feeling down or overwhelmed. Friends and loved ones will listen to your fears, hopes, and dreams and make you feel seen and understood. They can help you solve problems and think through alternatives, and they can distract you from your worries when that is what's really needed. In doing all this, they provide encouragement and lower your stress levels and feelings of loneliness.

The important thing is that you know the truth. This is all that matters, but be very careful who you let into your circle now. To achieve your best results in healing, it is paramount to involve as many healthy people as possible, even though it can feel like the exact opposite of what you want to do when you are first making these significant life and behavioral changes. You may lose family members as well as old friends when you start your journey of healing from narcissistic abuse, but know that this is common and that you are not alone.

Who do you trust to walk alongside you? Here are some ideas of who you can and should have on your team.

- A **Comforter** listens without judgment.
- A **Clarifier** supports our thinking by listening to and helping us work through our problems whenever we find ourselves stuck.
- A **Challenger** is someone who doesn't just tell us what we want to hear but gives us a no-nonsense reality check.
- A **Cheerleader** always celebrates our decisions and is quick to highlight that we are on the right path.

Our support system in life should be assembled thoughtfully. It's important to have the right support in place so that you actually have people who know what they are talking about to help you move forward! Wisdom, experience, and insight can be gained from friends, family, or colleagues who have been there and have learned what it takes to prevail, but be sure that these people are interested in your well-being. Start by educating yourself and others about what you need. For family and friends to understand what you're going through, they may need to learn more about narcissistic abuse. It's not always easy, but the first step is to have frank conversations about what you are going through and what you need from them to keep moving forward. I also recommend pointing your friends and family members to professional resources, such as books or websites run by licensed clinical therapists, as they will add some credence to what you're explaining to them.

Copy this list to a journal and fill it out; keep it handy so you know who to go to when you need support.

MY SUPPORT SYSTEM

Family members I am close to right now: _____

Friends I am in touch with right now: _____

Professionals in my life now (e.g., counselor, therapist, psychiatrist, life coach, lawyer): _____

Other support I have in my life right now: _____

Family members I would like to be close to in the future: _____

Friends I would like to be in touch with in the future (include people you may want to reconnect with): _____

Professionals I would like to have in the future (e.g., counselor, coach, therapist, psychiatrist, lawyer): _____

Other support I would like to have in the future: _____

Accountability buddies: _____

My work friend (support in your field is always good): _____

My counterpart (going through it also): _____

My cheerleader (always positive): _____

My realist (tells you the truth): _____

My fit friend (gets me moving): _____

Therapist: _____

WAYS YOU CAN EXPAND YOUR SUPPORT NETWORK

- Find people who share your interests. Cultivate new hobbies and network within those environments.
- Exercise. There is nothing like a good workout to stimulate your happy hormones (i.e., endorphins). The aftereffects can last up to three hours and put you in a positive frame of mind.
- Volunteer at an organization that shares your interests and values.

AVOID SURROUNDING YOURSELF WITH:

- People with whom the narcissist may have business connections
- People who are indebted to the narcissist
- People who are not willing to understand your pain
- Opportunistic people
- People who discount your experience
- People who try to hurry you into healing faster
- People who shame you for your experience
- People who victim-blame
- People who betray you

THE NARCISSIST'S FORMER SUPPLIES

You might assume that other survivors of a narcissist's abuse belong on the list of people to avoid, but think again! You may be the "caboose" on this train of misery and the train cars (people) before you may have tons of important information that could add value and clarity to your healing process. Be ready to accept your abuser's former sources of narcissist supply into your life. The benefits of doing so are many and varied.

- They understand exactly what you went through and can be extremely validating.
- They can hold space for you as you process difficult truths.
- They can fill in blanks that you may not understand.

- They can help strengthen any legal arguments you may need to make.
- They may have books and other resources that helped them connect the dots.
- They may have other friends and interpersonal resources to offer.
- They can also feel validated by hearing your story, so the relationship is mutually beneficial.

Many people feel concerned that they will look like a stalker or are overstepping their boundaries if they reach out to their narcissist's former sources of supply. This is so understandable, and many people will not want to hear from an ex that they think is jealous or out to hurt their relationship. Each scenario is different, so use caution here. Remember, though: The narcissist is lying about you, saying that you are a crazy, jealous, thirsty slut who is out to harm them, so might they not have done the same thing with their former supplies? (Categorically, the answer is yes!) They all do this, but I have found tremendous healing by connecting with my ex's former supplies. It changed my life. If you do not have success, this can feel like a barrier to your healing. You will find other ways to get validation, but you need to do it safely. Let's talk about ways to create a safe place to heal. Learning about boundaries and how to protect and care for yourself is crucial.

USE ASSERTIVE COMMUNICATION

This will not only help you form better relationships and find new opportunities, it can also shift the way you think about yourself and the way others view you. For women, this can prove very challenging because we live in a culture where we may be afraid that such a communication style will get us called a "bitch," but it is so important to realize that developing better, more assertive communication helps protect us from toxic people and from going through the trauma that the narcissistic breakup brings to us.

Further, we as codependents, people pleasers, and approval seekers need to learn how to set boundaries and how to trust our gut! Let's start with the often-expressed phrase "I am sorry." You may have learned to use this, even when it should be the other person saying it, as a form of protection to keep the other person from getting angry at you. You can say you are sorry for hurting someone's feelings, but you need to be aware of where the sorry is coming from. Is it to protect you from hurting someone's feelings, or is it because you mean it in earnest? We say we are sorry far too much, and taking the time to catch this is a terrific first step in developing boundaries. If you can curb your use of this phrase, you have taken the first step toward setting boundaries.

If you're having trouble differentiating assertive communication from other communication styles, here's a breakdown of some communication styles and how they impact our interpersonal lives.

- **Passive Communication:** Defined by being too nice or weak, overly compliant, avoiding eye contact, speaking softly, putting oneself down, being emotionally dishonest, and allowing others to trample you in conversation
- **Assertive Communication:** Defined by being firm but polite, compromising, maintaining warm and friendly eye contact and a conversational tone, building up others and oneself, being appropriately honest, and standing up for oneself
- **Aggressive Communication:** Defined by speaking in a mean, harsh, or sarcastic manner, taking instead of compromising, maintaining glaring eye contact and speaking in loud or threatening tones, putting others down, being inappropriately honest, and bullying or trampling others

Assertive communication is ideal because it allows you to express your opinions in an open, honest, and direct way. It allows you to take responsibility for yourself without judging or blaming others. Communicating assertively means expressing your ideas in a civilized way without being too aggressive or too passive. Passive is too nice, overly compliant, and weak. Assertive is firm but polite. Aggressive is mean, harsh, and sarcastic.

"I" STATEMENTS AND "YOU" STATEMENTS

In your daily life, you might have discovered a subtle difference between assertive and aggressive communication. Assertive communication is factual while aggressive communication is more judgmental and unfair to other people. What's more, aggressive communicators often jab a finger at you, using "you" statements during arguments.

EXAMPLES OF "YOU" STATEMENTS

"Why are you acting so mean to me?"
"Why are you being so nosy?"

The person's immediate reaction is to be defensive! Instead of being aggressive in this way, use "I" statements to discuss yourself and your feelings.

EXAMPLES OF "I" STATEMENTS

"I feel uncomfortable when you raise your voice to me."
"I do not feel comfortable sharing something so personal."

Using "I" statements takes practice and may feel a little foreign at first. Being able to keep the conversation on topic about your own feelings and needs will actually cause less arguing, though, and will keep the real issue at the forefront of the discussion! It can be difficult to prioritize yourself at first, but start to treat yourself as someone deserving of respect.

Give Yourself Permission. The biggest obstacle in asking for what you want is fear that someone will get mad or be disappointed. Make a conscious decision to prioritize what you want and be okay with that.

Be Specific About What You Want. When setting boundaries, be clear and concise. Avoid asking others to change.

Ask Without Apology. When you're setting a boundary, don't apologize. You have just as much right to have your boundaries recognized as the other person does to have their needs met.

Manage Your Expectations. Asking for what you want doesn't guarantee you will get it.

Accept the No. You will not always get what you want. Know that the "win" is in the asking, not in the receiving.

EXAMPLES OF HEALTHY BOUNDARIES

Need a better idea of how you might set a healthy boundary? Here are two concrete examples to consider before you try to establish your own.

> "I don't like to talk on the phone during work hours, so when I'm at work I don't accept personal calls until after five p.m. If you try to contact me, I will not answer until after five o'clock."

> "In my relationship, I value and expect monogamy, quality time each week (so at least one date night a week), and 100 percent honesty at all times. I will not stay in a relationship that doesn't have this basic foundation."

It is impossible to set boundaries without also setting consequences, but make sure those consequences are realistic and doable. If you are setting boundaries in a relationship and you are not yet at a point where you are ready to leave the relationship, then don't say that you will leave if your boundaries go unacknowledged. Never create a consequence on which you are not willing to follow through. To set boundaries and not enforce them just gives the other person an excuse to continue with the same old behavior.

For an example of a consequence you should be able to follow through on, you might say: "If you call me names, I will confront you about your behavior each and every time, and will share my feelings with you. I will not tolerate verbal abuse. If you continue this behavior, I will weigh my options, including leaving this relationship. I do not deserve this, and I will not put up with it any longer."

SELF-CARE

As you recover from narcissistic abuse, there are going to be a lot of draining days. Whether it's facing your ex and their legal team in the courtroom, dealing with former friends who "don't believe you," or merely learning how to live on your own again, this necessary healing process can take a lot out of you. This is why creating a safe place for yourself cannot happen without self-care, a concept pioneered by Black activist Angela Davis in the 1970s.

Self-care includes nourishment, sleep hygiene, and hydration as well as spending time with people we care for and working on our goals. Self-care also includes paying attention to our immune system by lowering stress and worrying less.

Each time you fly on a plane, you're reminded that, in the event of an emergency, you should put your oxygen mask on before you attempt to put one on anyone else. When you give yourself time each day to focus on taking care of yourself, it will be easier to accomplish all the other things that you need to each day, especially caring for your children.

Many of us who were in toxic relationships focused so much attention on our worries that we were too exhausted to do much of anything else. This is not healthy. It is time to focus on *you*! Many of us who have experienced trauma need to lean into a radical self-love phase, whether it's taking fifteen minutes in the morning to stretch, making yourself a cup of tea or cocoa, or getting away for a few hours or a weekend.

In your journal, or on your laptop or phone, spend some time answering the following question. Once you have established five self-care practices, schedule them into your calendar as you would a doctor's visit or any other essential appointment.

What Are Some Ways I Can Practice Self-Love?

1. _____

2. _____

3. _____

4. _____

5. _____

LIMITING BELIEFS

Another critical barrier to recovery is the concept of limiting beliefs, especially those we hold about ourselves and what we are capable of. You may think that you are not young enough or smart enough or valued enough. You may have had a parent tell you that you are not ever going to be successful or a bully in school that called you "fat" or "a loser." Even social media makes so many people feel that they need to live up to some unrealistic expectation of success. Limiting beliefs are not adding value to anyone.

EMPOWERING BELIEFS

Here's an exercise to help you start shifting your cognition to empowering beliefs. For every limiting belief that comes to your mind, figure out a way to change it around to make it more positive. Set a timer for fifteen minutes and journal the following:

Limiting Belief: I don't have enough education.

Empowering Belief: I can go back to school to achieve my goals.

Limiting Belief: _____

Empowering Belief: _____

Limiting Belief: _____

Empowering Belief: _____

Limiting Belief: _____

Empowering Belief: _____

Limiting Belief: _____

Empowering Belief: _____

How did it feel to shift away from your limiting beliefs? Were you able to do it? Thinking positively can feel uncomfortable at first, especially if you've primarily been thinking in terms of limiting beliefs, but if you stick with it, your growth will be remarkable. What did you learn about yourself and the way you think about yourself? Did you find that it added value to think more positively? If so, then you will really like the upcoming section on positive affirmations.

POSITIVE AFFIRMATIONS

Positive affirmations are designed to encourage an optimistic mind-set and have been shown to help with the tendency to linger on negative experiences or ruminate about what we've been through, which is what many do after an abusive relationship. You might think this is thinly disguised "toxic positivity," but we are not looking to create some false Hallmark movie scenario. Positive affirmations aim to get you to a place of improved self-esteem. The narcissist worked systematically to break yours down, potentially so far down that you cannot find your way out of it. Building self-esteem is so important to your healing from narcissistic abuse, and you can do so through regular reminders of how much you love, care for, and respect yourself. High self-esteem boosts mental well-being, helps you handle adversity in a positive manner, and helps you develop healthy coping skills.

POSITIVE AFFIRMATIONS

Use the following guidance to build some positive affirmations of your own.

- Affirmations often start with the words "I am" and are always positively phrased. This means you should never use a negative word in an affirmation. For example, instead of writing, "I am not afraid of public speaking," you could write, "I am a confident public speaker."
- Affirmations are short and specific. Instead of writing, "I am driving a new car," you could write, "I am driving a new Porsche."
- Affirmations are in the present tense and often include an action word.
- Affirmations have a "feeling" word in them. Examples of this include "confidently," "successfully," or "gracefully."
- Affirmations are about you and should be about your own behavior, never someone else's.
- Say and visualize your affirmations every day.
- Here are some examples of good affirmations:

"I am safe."

"I deserve to love myself and be loved by others."

"I am unique. I feel good about being alive and being me."

"I am okay as I am and I accept and love myself."

"I inhale love and exhale fear."

"I have unlimited power at my disposal."

"I matter, and what I have to offer this world matters."

ADDRESS NEGATIVE AUTOMATIC
THOUGHTS AND SELF-TALK

In a similar way to working with limiting versus empowering beliefs, and positive thinking, the following exercise is a great way to address negative automatic thoughts and self-talk—common problems that people with low self-esteem or mental health issues face. Challenging negative self-talk is a core technique in cognitive behavioral therapy (CBT), which has proven effective in a wide range of conditions, diagnoses, and problems.

CHALLENGING NEGATIVE SELF-TALK

This exercise will help you work on changing negative cognition.
Trigger—Write down what prompted your negative thought. (If any of these thoughts become too much, always pace yourself.) Think back to the moment the negative thought first popped into your head and write down whatever immediately preceded it.

Negative Thought—Write down the negative thought.

Associated Emotion—Now, think about the emotions that arise when you say the negative thought out loud. Whether it's anger, sadness, guilt, disgust, or another emotion entirely, write down whatever feelings are provoked by voicing the negative thought.

Evidence That Does Not Support the Thought—This is where you must think hard about the negative thought and decide how well it truly applies to you. For example, you may have gotten some disappointing feedback from your boss on a report you handed in, but if you're thinking, "I'm a failure at everything," you have fallen prey to taking a single incident and overgeneralizing.

_____

_____

Alternative Thought—Reflect on the thought and come up with a thought that you believe to replace it. This thought should be more in line with the truth, but with a positive message and data that supports it. If the original negative thought was "I am fat," then the alternative thought has to be something you actually believe and have data to prove, so if "I am skinny" doesn't feel like something you believe, try "I am strong."

_____

_____

Associated Emotion—The alternative thought should make you feel a better emotion than the original negative thought did.

_____

This first exercise is a good one to help you get used to the mindful sort of thinking that cognitive behavioral therapy (CBT) encourages. So, too, are the handful of exercises that follow.

FIVE THINGS YOU LIKE ABOUT YOURSELF

We all have negative cognition that may have developed when we were children that becomes our inner dialogue. Many women have it regarding their appearance, and many men have it around their ability to make money or have a successful career. We need to combat this inner critic with countered, logical responses.

If I have a girl in my head who tells me that I am unlovable all day because I used to get bullied, then I need to develop counterresponses, such as "No. I am worthy." They have to be statements that you believe. If you have to use "I am working on it," that can be enough of a counterresponse (as long as you are taking steps to work on it). Remember, you have to be able to believe the new statement. Be careful here. *Don't* use statements that are contingent upon another's experience of you, such as "caring" or "generous." Think of yourself and yourself alone. I don't care if the statement is "I have a nice ass." It has to be about *you*.

————— ∞∞∞ —————

In your journal, list five things you like about yourself.

1. _____

2. _____

3. _____

4. _____

5. _____

COMMON CLICHÉS

Cognitive behavioral therapy can even help you deprogram from the ways in which the narcissist wanted you to think. For instance, the narcissist wants you to live in "Confusion Land," so they often use clichés to keep you rooted in the untruths they've cultivated in your mind. These clichés work so well to perplex us because they are embedded in the language of everyday conversation. In other words, by attaching their lies to phrases you've heard so often that you accept them at face value, the narcissist makes it easier to accept their lies at face value.

There are a lot of outside influences that impact how we feel, what we do, and, most of all, what we believe. These may include very common limiting belief systems that are passed from generation to generation and person to person via clichés. A lot of the work we have to do after narcissistic abuse involves taking the time to check our cognition and develop new pathways in our mind. To do this, we must become aware of which thoughts we have and then question them. When we question a belief, we can often find evidence to the contrary, which weakens our acceptance of it. Consider these clichés:

- "Think outside the box."
- "There's no 'I' in team."
- "Tomorrow is another day."
- "Better late than never."
- "Love is blind."
- "All is fair in love and war."
- "Don't burn your bridges."
- "Good things come to those who wait."
- "Let go of the past." (*The narcissist loves this one.*)
- "No pain, no gain."
- "Life is hard."
- "Relationships are hard work."
- "You have to pay your dues."

In your journal, answer these questions:

Which of these phrases were you conditioned to believe?

Can you see any fears you developed because of them?

GRATITUDE JOURNALING

It seems that gratitude journaling is everywhere—and maybe that makes you roll your eyes. But trust me, another great cognitive behavioral therapeutic practice is to journal and shift your perspective to one of gratitude.

A gratitude journal is a tool to keep track of the good things in life and truly consider the things you are really grateful for. No matter how difficult and defeating life can sometimes feel, there is always something to feel grateful for. While it can be tough to find something to be grateful for in a rough patch, doing so can actually help pull you out of your funk. More than that, regularly journaling about the good things in your life can help prepare and strengthen you to deal with the rough patches when they pop up.

Here are a few benefits people have noticed once they started practice gratitude journaling:

- It lowers stress levels.
- It can help you feel calmer, especially at night.
- Journaling can give you a new perspective on what is important to you and what you truly appreciate in your life.
- By noting what you are grateful for, you can gain clarity on what you want to have more of in your life and what you can do without.
- Keeping a gratitude journal helps you learn more about yourself and become more self-aware.
- Your gratitude journal is for your eyes only, so you can write anything you feel without worrying about judgment from others.
- On days when you feel blue, you can read through your gratitude journal to readjust your attitude and remember all the good things in your life.

GRATEFUL

It's simple to start: just write down the things you are grateful for on a daily basis. You can use a journal, a diary, a notebook, a piece of paper, or log it in your phone. Once you have your journal or app ready, start noting the things you are grateful for, and anytime you reach a goal or receive good news, journal about it.

Let's try it now; grab your journal and record the following:

What are you grateful for?

1. _____
2. _____
3. _____
4. _____
5. _____

BREATHING

As a therapist, I am required to take continuing education classes to maintain my license. In all the continuing education credits that I have ever taken, a fair number have involved learning breathing techniques, but I never felt connected to this form of coping or meditative practice until I remembered some of the ways that I would calm myself before an Ironman race. (And I think it's fair to say that removing yourself from a narcissistic relationship has a lot in common with an endurance race!)

At the beginning of this large triathlon, I would be very nervous. People will often kick you or swim over you during the swimming portion of the race, and it can feel scary. To get myself to relax in the face of that threat, I would focus on my exhale, just breathing out slowly. People innately breathe in quickly when they are scared or nervous, so paying close attention to the exhale instead of the inhale proves to be very helpful to me to calm myself.

If, like me, you've wanted to get into a breathwork practice but have struggled in the past to do so, I would recommend learning to breathe slowly and focusing on the exhale whenever you're dealing with any of the stresses that life throws our way. You can start simply: inhale for a count of six, and exhale for a count of six, whenever you feel you need a break or to reset yourself.

WORKING ON SELF-ACTUALIZATION

I've talked about self-actualization a few times throughout this book—and with good reason. Working toward self-actualization can take a lifetime, so give yourself grace. Here are some ideas that can help you best conceptualize this path and what it will take to get you the best results.

Passions

Rediscovering your passions and inspirations is another huge part of the healing process. It's also a good way to identify self-care practices that work for you and self-actualization avenues that resonate with you. After all, to some people, running a marathon sounds like a blast; to others, it sounds like a great way to spend $200 to not be able to walk by the end of the day.

Once you start learning what you love and following what feels good, you will be less and less attracted to what doesn't feel good anymore. Looking to have more passion in our daily lives keeps us from interacting with anyone or anything that takes time away from it. The goal of the following exercise is to uncover something about yourself, something new perhaps, or something forgotten. If you love it, keep doing it, or if you are curious about a new endeavor you've always wanted to try, go for it. Step outside your comfort zone! I recommend making a list of the ones you think you have interest in but make that list robust.

READ THROUGH THE FOLLOWING LIST

1. Soaking in the bathtub
2. Planning my career
3. Collecting things (coins, shells, etc.)
4. Going on vacation
5. Thinking how it will be when I finish school
6. Recycling old items
7. Going to a movie in the middle of the week
8. Jogging, walking
9. Buying household gadgets
10. Lying in the sun
11. Planning a career change
12. Listening to others
13. Reading magazines or newspapers
14. Hobbies (stamp collecting, model building, etc.)
15. Spending an evening with good friends
16. Planning a day's activities
17. Meeting new people
18. Remembering beautiful scenery
19. Saving money
20. Going home from work
21. Practicing karate, judo, yoga
22. Thinking about retirement
23. Repairing things around the house
24. Working on my car (bicycle)
25. Remembering the words and deeds of loving people
26. Having quiet evenings
27. Taking care of my plants
28. Buying, selling stock
29. Going swimming
30. Doodling
31. Exercising
32. Collecting old things
33. Going to a party
34. Playing golf
35. Playing soccer
36. Flying kites
37. Having discussions with friends
38. Having family get-togethers
39. Riding a motorbike
40. Running a track
41. Going camping
42. Singing around the house
43. Arranging flowers
44. Going to the beach
45. A day with nothing to do
46. Going skating
47. Going sailing
48. Painting
49. Doing needlepoint
50. Playing musical instruments
51. Doing arts and crafts
52. Making a gift for someone
53. Cooking
54. Going hiking
55. Writing (stories, poems, articles)
56. Working
57. Sightseeing
58. Gardening
59. Playing tennis
60. Going to plays and concerts
61. Going for a drive
62. Refinishing furniture
63. Going bike riding

64. Walks in the woods
65. Walks on the beach or at the waterfront
66. Buying gifts
67. Traveling to national parks
68. Completing a task
69. Collecting shells
70. Going to a spectator sport (auto racing, horse racing)
71. Teaching
72. Photography
73. Going fishing
74. Thinking about pleasant events
75. Playing with animals
76. Reading fiction
77. Acting
78. Being alone
79. Writing diary entries or letters
80. Cleaning
81. Reading nonfiction
82. Taking children places
83. Dancing
84. Going on a picnic
85. Meditating
86. Playing volleyball or any team sport
87. Having lunch with a friend
88. Going to the mountains
89. Thinking about happy moments in my childhood
90. Playing cards
91. Playing guitar
92. Shooting pool
93. Going to museums
94. Getting a massage
95. Taking a sauna or a steam bath
96. Going skiing
97. White-water canoeing
98. Going bowling
99. Going horseback riding

Now, look at the things you wrote down. List five new hobbies you would like to try, then pick one or two and make notes for how you can make this happen.

1. _____
2. _____
3. _____
4. _____
5. _____

Moving Forward as You Heal

Once you've achieved some self-actualization and you feel ready to start tackling your healing journey, I'd like to offer up some exciting, alternate perspectives that may feel better to imagine, especially regarding dating and finances.

RETHINKING RELATIONSHIPS

In our society, there are lots of negative words used for women who are single and a lot of chatter that anyone who is single after a certain age is "too picky" or that there is something wrong with them. Being pushed toward marriage based on cultural norms and even movies and love songs happens without us even realizing it, but being single is amazing! You get to do what you want when you want, and it is all about *you*. Take this time to think about yourself and what you want the rest of your life to look like. Enjoy the freedom!

You may realize after this experience that you dated more than one narcissist so it can be scary to reenter the dating world. If and when you do decide to date again, I have a couple of tested and proven pieces of advice to share with you. I don't subscribe to the "take it slow" perspective, especially when it comes to telling a new partner about your past or establishing boundaries. Instead, I recommend setting boundaries early, so as to not waste time. Additionally:

- See how your new partner responds to your doing your own things, such as practicing self-care or staying involved in your own hobbies.
- Watch how they respond to your excelling in your career or another endeavor—the narcissist or toxic person will not want you to do well in your career. If they come to learn that you are "leveling up," they may lash out or try to undermine you. Pay close attention to how they respond to your accolades, especially if they are braggarts and/or try to one-up your accomplishments or belittle them.
- Do they talk about themselves a lot and make themselves sound better than they really are?

- Be mindful that narcissists are masters at pretending to be real, but they will also exhibit subtle inconsistencies in what they say and do.
- It is a red flag if they are talking about superficial things, such as money, cars, Rolexes, or anything like that.
- Look to see if they are unkind to the waitstaff. Many narcissists behave as if they are superior to others.

It is self-care to make your boundaries known early on. See how they respond when you make mistakes. Take the wrong exit when you are late to something that they are looking forward to, and gauge their reaction. Many think that this approach is radical, but your safety is at risk here, so be wise and keep on the lookout for red flags.

You now have the skills, if you choose to use them, to look for these signs very early on and protect yourself.

Bottom line: I do not fundamentally agree with taking things slow because that is exactly what the narcissist can count on, even if it looks like they are trying to move fast. It is the slow, toxic fumes that seep in over time that do the most damage. Be firm in your boundaries and be prepared to move on if you are pushed in a way that makes you uncomfortable or feels unsafe. While it may sound harsh, I also recommend not giving the benefit of the doubt on anything. Your sovereignty depends on it. Seek authenticity, vulnerability, and depth. That's where love lives.

GOAL-SETTING

After you've begun to feel stable in your life after abuse, you may feel independent and safe enough to establish new goals for yourself. This section can help walk you through it.

A goal is a statement of an end result, to be achieved in a specified period of time at a specific level of quality. In short, it should be *measurable*. When we are creating goals, we need to be specific. Too often, we say we are going to do too much too quickly, and when we don't succeed, we add that to "our list of failures" and tell ourselves that we *can't*, when the bigger reality is that we just didn't set the right goals. If you find yourself having trouble setting goals—and many of us who are survivors do—here are some things to help you set SMART goals. If you have a goal, but find that fears are in the way, looking at your goal through the SMART lens can help it become more attainable.

A "SMART" goal is:

Specific. What do you want to accomplish? What, exactly, do you want to do? Who is involved? What may be the barriers to success? Why do it?

Measurable. You need to be able to track your progress. Choose a unit of measurement as well as the target amount you'll consider a success.

Achievable. Be realistic. Is it within your capability and control? Losing 10 pounds in three months is achievable, whereas losing 10 pounds in three days is not.

Relevant. Your goal should be important to you. Is it in-line with your personal vision?

Time-Bound. When do you want to accomplish your goal? Select a date in the future. When will it be completed?

Having an action plan will make goals happen. A good action plan sets the stage for achieving the goal; it maps out the process with a detailed schedule of key activities needed to accomplish small goals so as to connect the dots and achieve the bigger goal you are envisioning. Break down the bigger goal into smaller goals; they can be broken down into daily, weekly, monthly, and yearly installments. Determine the resources that are required to achieve each one. Identify who you will need to coordinate with and who you will rely on to contribute. Anticipate problems and outline contingency plans.

Clarify your *big* goal. What does the expected outcome look like? How will you know whether you have reached your destination? What makes your goal measurable? What constraints do you have, such as limits on time, money, or other resources?

Write a list of actions. Write down all the actions you may need to take to achieve your goal. Write down as many different options and ideas as possible.

Organize your list into a plan. Decide on the order of your action steps. Start by looking at what is the most important, and go from there. For each action, what other steps should be completed before that action? Write down one to three goals and work toward them.

CREATE A VISION BOARD

The more we can visualize our goals, the greater chance we have of accomplishing them. Take what you have learned throughout this entire process and create a board that will inspire you each day to keep moving forward.

- Buy a large piece of poster board or use any material that you like.
- Use old magazines, photos, newspapers, paint, markers.
- Include pictures, phrases, stories, and artwork that will inspire you.
- Start by focusing on what you want the next year of your life to look like:
  » Travel
  » Work or education
  » Family
  » Personal care

Be creative! Boards can be as big as you want. When you are finished, make sure to place it somewhere you can see it every day. You will be amazed what you can manifest when you have a visual of what you are working toward!

———— ∞ ————

As we near the end of this book, I want to wish you congratulations for staying true to yourself and putting in the work. You have been through an extremely dark and challenging period, but likely, life has already started to take you in a more positive direction than you have been in a long time (if ever!). Don't think you are alone and damaged. You can be dealing with trauma AND also living your best life. You can be thriving AND surviving; scared AND empowered. Survivors are many things at once. These things are not mutually exclusive.

Your power has always been within you. Perhaps that's something you're beginning to realize. You are strong, smart, caring, and, most of all, worthy. Let the confusion go and trust yourself. All those small whispers of "something is wrong" that you heard along the way were right, and you dodged a bullet! No matter how long you were with your abuser and how many mistakes you made along the way, whenever you get away from the narcissist, you are the victor—you win! All the nights that you cried yourself to sleep will slowly vanish. All the lies are exposed now, and you are free to move forward with your life. The mask is off, and you can now see clearly what has happened and become the person you were destined to be.

Give yourself grace. You have gone through a significant trauma and deserve to take your time to heal. Your future self is so proud of what you are doing to stay free from further abuse. Your ancestors are so proud of you and what you are doing to heal! If you have children, they are going to be proud of what you are doing to break the cycle and live in the truth.

Ignore the jerks in your life who believe your abuser. It takes a special person to go through what you have endured and still keep going. If you were to blink your eyes and wake up four years from now, you would be smiling and breathing easy, knowing that you did the right thing. Time helps, and you will see that staying would have been a mistake. You will see that the narcissist ends up doing the same thing to their next supply.

I am so proud of you, and I am right by your side. Take these tools and use them to create whatever life you desire and deserve. Working on your goals, taking daily action steps, and having the right people on your team will ensure your success. The future is yours . . . and remember, I cannot keep narcissists from coming for your energy, but I have cracked the code on how to make them go away fast. Stick close to the things that actually matter—yourself, your friends, your finances, your career, and your hobbies—and narcissists will move on. They are allergic to your autonomy, so always stay close to those things and you will have success. Stay passionately, intensely, lovingly, and devotedly attached to your essence. When you get away, you are the victor. As Lauryn Hill says, "How you gonna win when you ain't right within?" They are not right within and you are. You win. Never give up on the truth, and never give up on yourself. You are your own superpower.

Glossary

Attachment Styles:

Anxious Attachment. People with this attachment style may experience intense emotional discomfort or avoidance of being alone, have difficulty setting boundaries and trusting others, experience fear of abandonment, feel that they are unworthy of love, but also have an intense desire for intimacy or closeness.

Avoidant Attachment. Avoidant attachment starts when a parent doesn't show care or responsiveness past providing essentials, such as food and shelter. The child disregards their own needs to maintain peace and keep their caregiver close by. They tend to be very independent and have few emotional connections with others.

Disorganized Attachment. People with this attachment style develop it from a childhood of dealing with a neglectful or abusive primary caregiver. This style manifests itself as people who find intimate relationships confusing and unsettling or swing between feelings for their partner of extreme love and extreme hate. They can be insensitive, selfish, and controlling with an overarching theme of unworthiness.

Secure Attachment. People with this attachment style tend to be empathetic and able to set appropriate boundaries, They tend to feel safe, stable, and more satisfied in their close relationships. They don't fear being on their own and they usually thrive in close, meaningful relationships.

Breadcrumbing. Also called Hansel and Greteling, breadcrumbing is a colloquial term used to characterize the practice of sporadically feigning interest in another person so as to keep them interested, despite a true lack of investment in the relationship.

Capture-Bonding, a.k.a. Stockholm Syndrome. A victim has a psychological response, sometimes seen in an abducted hostage, whereby the hostage shows signs of loyalty to the hostage taker. Victims of narcissistic abuse will flex their "justification muscle," making excuses for their abusers because of the cognitive dissonance or confusion they are feeling about the different versions of the person they are bonded to. In many cases, because of this trauma bond, they may even defend them or aid them in harming others.

Codependency. A dysfunctional relationship dynamic where one person assumes the role of "the giver," sacrificing their own needs and well-being for the sake of the other, "the taker." Codependent people are often approval seekers and people pleasers.

Coercive Control. An act or a pattern of acts of threats, humiliation, and intimidation or other abuse that is used to harm, punish, or frighten their victim. This is a hallmark of narcissistic abuse and domestic violence.

Cognitive Behavioral Therapy (CBT). A form of psychological treatment that has been demonstrated to be effective for a range of problems, including depression and anxiety disorders, whereby there is a conscious shift in cognition.

Cognitive Dissonance. The experience of having two competing thoughts at the same time or holding conflicting beliefs, thoughts, and values.

Confabulation. When a disordered person generates a false memory. It differs from delusions, in that delusions are false beliefs and confabulations are false memories. Narcissists that confabulate may fill in the blanks of their memories with fake stories to embellish or brag.

Core Wound. A deep emotional wound formed and internalized from a significant event in childhood.

Dialectical Behavioral Therapy (DBT). An evidence-based psychotherapy that focuses on helping people accept the reality of their lives and their behaviors, as well as helping them learn to change their lives through mindfulness, stress tolerance, emotional regulation, and interpersonal effectiveness.

Dissociation. A break in how the mind handles information, including a feeling of disconnection from thoughts, feelings, memories, and surroundings and even on one's sense of identity and perception of time.

Flying Monkeys. The minions or enablers of the narcissist, who aid and abet the abuser but are, themselves, sometimes unknowingly under coercion. They can be family, friends, colleagues, or on a grander scale, lawyers, therapists, or politicians.

Future-Faking. This term refers to "dangling a carrot" when a toxic person promises something to manipulate a victim into giving them something they want, but not delivering on what they promised.

Gaslighting. An insidious form of manipulation and psychological control whereby victims are deliberately and systematically fed false information that leads them to question the truth. Some can end up doubting their memory, their perception, and even their sanity.

Golden Child. A child of narcissistic parent(s) who usually are controlling and authoritarian. The golden child is the one that the narcissist projects onto the most and gets the best treatment. The narcissist will oftentimes groom this child to be somewhat of an extension of the toxic parent, and it may manifest itself in the narcissistic parent's making a "mini-me" by pushing them to play sports or do other things that the toxic parent likes to do.

Hoovering. This is a manipulative tactic that a narcissist uses to lure a person back into the relationship.

Intermittent Reinforcement. Psychologist B. F. Skinner discovered that while behavior is often influenced by rewards or punishment, there is a specific way rewards are doled out that can cause that behavior to persist over long periods of time, causing that behavior to become less vulnerable to extinction.

Lost Child. The invisible one that tries to stay quiet, because the narcissistic parent is so busy building up their golden child or tormenting other people in the family that the lost child is forgotten. They will be left on their own with no parental guidance and may have to raise themselves. Many end up being loners in their adult life and may experience challenges in developing interpersonal relationships.

Love-Bombing. Also known as "idealization," love-bombing is the over-the-top gift giving and adulation that comes in front of a devalue stage used by a toxic person to manipulate victims into subscribing to the narcissist's false persona.

Luring. Luring by the narcissist includes the stalking, love-bombing, and hoovering behaviors whereby they are fixated on gaining your trust and manipulating you into their false reality.

Machiavellian. A personality trait that denotes cunningness, the ability to be manipulative, to use whatever means necessary to gain power, status and money. Machiavellianism is one of the traits that forms the Dark Triad, along with narcissism and psychopathy.

Mirroring. A manipulation tactic used by narcissistic individuals to create a false sense of connection with another person by mimicking their thoughts, feelings, interests, or behaviors.

Narcissistic Collapse. When a narcissist believes that someone is threatening their ability to maintain their superficial inflated ego or their fragile self-esteem is damaged, it can result in intense reactions and abuse toward others. Instead of reflecting on what happened or trying to address the conflict appropriately, they can become hysterical, volatile, or rageful toward themselves or those around them.

Narcissistic Entitlement. A narcissist might believe they are extraordinary or exceptionally deprived and therefore deserve to be treated better than they are, or they simply feel superior and feel they deserve the best. In either case, the rules that apply to everyone else don't apply to them. The narcissist owes the world nothing while the world owes them everything.

Narcissistic Personality Disorder (NPD). Narcissistic personality disorder involves a pattern of self-centered, arrogant thinking and behavior, a lack of empathy and consideration for other people, with an excessive need for admiration. People with NPD are described as cocky, manipulative, selfish, patronizing, and demanding.

Postseparation Abuse. This abuse is characterized by an ongoing campaign to maintain power and control over anyone bold enough to extricate themselves from a cult or abusive relationship or who is pushed out of the relationship. It shows up via courtroom legal abuse, threats and intimidation, smear campaigns, and the exploitation of children or collateral gathered during the relationship.

Scapegoat Child. The scapegoat child embodies what the narcissistic parent cannot stand in themselves. By projecting what they hate in themselves onto the scapegoat child, the parent feels better about themselves.

Shared Psychotic Disorder. This is a rare disorder characterized by sharing a delusion among two or more people in a close relationship. The narcissist who has a psychotic disorder with delusions influences one or more nonpsychotic individuals to believe this delusion.

Silent Treatment. A form of emotional abuse or manipulation whereby one person ignores or refuses to engage with another person as a way to exert control or punishment. It can be used to make the other person feel anxious, isolated, or guilty.

Smear Campaign. An effort to damage or call into question someone's reputation by propounding negative propaganda.

Sociopathy. Also called antisocial personality disorder (APD), refers to a condition whereby a person consistently shows no regard for right and wrong and ignores the rights and feelings of others. It is often characterized by a lack of empathy, criminality, impulsive behavior, aggression, not learning from mistakes, lying, physical violence, enjoying other people's suffering, drug abuse, irresponsibility, and overall risky/hazardous behavior.

Stonewalling. A refusal to communicate or cooperate. This behavior occurs in such situations as trying to mediate in court proceedings with a narcissist.

Supply (Narcissistic Supply). The constant supply of attention and admiration needed by narcissists. To gain this attention, narcissists often use a "false self" that is likable to attract people to them.

Trauma Bond. When a person forms a deep emotional attachment with someone that causes them harm. It often develops from a repeated cycle of abuse and positive reinforcement. It can feel like codependency or addiction to the abuser.

Triangulation. A technique commonly used by the narcissist to create drama and tension between two people to enable the narcissist to maintain control and feel superior.

Withholding. Refusing to give affection and information as a form of punishment. Withholding causes victims to attempt to please the narcissist so as to regain the initial attention and affection they experienced in the beginning of the relationship.

Notes

CHAPTER 1: THE MOST IMPORTANT THING: YOUR SAFETY

1. *Diagnostic and Statistical Manual of Mental Disorders*, 5th ed. (Washington, DC, American Psychiatric Association, 1968).
2. Frederick S. Stinson, Deborah A. Dawson, Rise B. Goldstein, et al., "Prevalence, Correlates, Disability, and Comorbidity of DSM-IV Narcissistic Personality Disorder: Results from the Wave 2 National Epidemiologic Survey on Alcohol and Related Conditions," *Journal of Clinical Psychiatry* 69, no. 7 (2008): 1033–1045, https://www.ncbi.nlm.nih.gov/pmc/articles/PMC2669224/.
3. Ramani Durvasula, "The Narcissism Doctor: '1 In 6 People Are Narcissists!' How to Spot Them & Can They Change?" podcast, March 2, 2024, https://www.youtube.com/watch?v=hTkKXDvSJvo.
4. Susanne Schade, "The Emotional Heritage of Postwar Germany: The Transgenerational Transmission of a Guilt Conflict," March 26, 2021, https://onlinelibrary.wiley.com/doi/10.1002/ppi.1587.
5. Saul McLeod, "Maslow's Hierarchy of Needs," Simply Psychology, January 24, 2024, https://www.simplypsychology.org/maslow.html.
6. Rebekah Sosa, "Maslow's Hierarchy of Needs," Medium.com, October 24, 2017, https://medium.com/re-write/maslows-hierarchy-of-needs-9ead9a46cb14.

CHAPTER 2: THE NARCISSIST'S CALLING CARDS

1. Mary Kowalchyk, Helena Palmieri, Elena Conte, et al., "Narcissism Through the Lens of Performative Self-Elevation," *Personality and Individual Differences* 177 (July 2021): 110780, https://www.sciencedirect.com/science/article/pii/S0191886921001550.
2. S. Ash, Dara Greenwood, and Julian Paul Keenan, "The Neural Correlates of Narcissism: Is There a Connection with Desire for Fame and Celebrity Worship," *Brain Sciences* 13, no. 10 (October 13, 2023): 1499, https://www.ncbi.nlm.nih.gov/pmc/articles/PMC10605183.

CHAPTER 3: EMPATHY NOT INCLUDED

1. *Diagnostic and Statistical Manual of Mental Disorders*, 5th ed. (Washington, DC, American Psychiatric Association, 1968).

2. Igor Nenadić, Carsten Lorenz, and Christian Gaser, "Narcissistic Personality Traits and Prefrontal Brain Structure," *Scientific Reports*, no. 15707 (August 3, 2021), https://www.nature.com/articles/s41598 -021-94920-z.

3. Greta Urbonaviciute, "Do Narcissists Lack Empathy? It Depends," SPSP (blog), November 19, 2021, https://spsp.org/news-center /character-context-blog/do-narcissists-lack-empathy-it-depends.

4. Miranda Giacomin, Christopher Brinton, and Nicholas O. Rule, "Narcissistic Individuals Exhibit Poor Recognition Memory," *Journal of Personality* 90, no. 5 (November 30, 2021): 675–689, https://pubmed.ncbi.nlm .nih.gov/34797571.

5. Kendra Cherry, "How to Know when You Love Someone," Very Well Mind, February 6, 2024, https://www.verywellmind.com/what-is -love-2795343.

6. Tom Neal, "To Will the Good of Another," Word of Fire, February 24, 2016, https://www.wordonfire.org/articles/to-will-the-good-of-the-other/.

7. Erich Fromm, "The Art of Loving," Artysana (blog), February 12, 2021, https://www.aartysana.com/blog/theartoflovingerichfromm.

8. Kristi A. Chin, "The Dark Side of Jealousy," April 8, 2016, https://ir.lib .uwo.ca/etd/3760/.

9. Gregory K. Totoriello, William Hart, Kyle Richardson, et al., "Do Narcissists Try to Make Romantic Partners Jealous on Purpose? An Examination of Motives for Deliberate Jealousy-Induction Among Subtypes of Narcissism," *Personality and Individual Differences* 114 (August 1, 2017): 10–15, https://www.sciencedirect.com/science/article/abs/pii /S0191886917302222.

10. Jeff Berkovici, "Why (Some) Psychopaths Make Great CEOs," *Forbes*, June 14, 2011, https://www.forbes.com/sites/jeffbercovici/2011/06/14 /why-some-psychopaths-make-great-ceos/; Jonathan Ronson, *The Psychopath Test: A Journey Through the Madness Industry* (New York: Riverhead Books, 2012).

11. Jody Schulz, "Stressed? Peppermint Can Help!" College of Agriculture & Natural Resources, Michigan State University, June 1, 2016, https: //www.canr.msu.edu/news/stressed_peppermint_can_help.

CHAPTER 4: WHAT THE NARCISSIST WILL NOT DO

1. Erica N. Carlson, Simine Vazire, and Thomas F. Oltmanns, "You Probably Think This Paper's About You: Narcissists' Perceptions of Their Personality and Reputation," *Journal of Personality and Social Psychology* 101, no. 1 (July 2012): 185–201, https://www.ncbi.nlm.nih.gov/pmc/articles/PMC3119754/.

CHAPTER 5: A CULT OF ONE

1. Robert J. Lifton, "Lifton's 'Cult Formation' with Commentary," Pairadocks (blog), February 1981, https://pairadocks.blogspot.com/2018/02/liftons-cult-formation-1981-with.html.
2. Julia Naftolin, "The 3 Main Personality Traits of Cult Leaders, According to a Cult-Recovery Therapist," Business Insider, September 24, 2020, https://www.businessinsider.com/3-cult-leader-types-says-therapist-treating-former-followers-2020-9.
3. Frank Parlato, "Keith Raniere Admits He Is a Psychopath in Shocking 2007 Article in Spanish Magazine," Frank Report, November 10, 2019, https://frankreport.com/2019/11/10/keith-raniere-admits-he-is-a-psychopath-in-shocking-2007-article-in-spanish-magazine/.
4. Naftolin, "The 3 Main Personality Traits."
5. Feras Al Saif and Yasir Al Khalili, *Shared Psychotic Disorder* (Treasure Island, FL: StatPearls Publishing, 2024), https://pubmed.ncbi.nlm.nih.gov/31095356.
6. Naftolin, "The 3 Main Personality Traits."
7. Leah Remini, *Troublemaker: Surviving Hollywood and Scientology* (New York: Ballantine Books, 2015).

CHAPTER 6: LIVING WITH A NARCISSIST

1. Women Against Abuse, "Why It's So Difficult to Leave," 2024, https://www.womenagainstabuse.org/education-resources/learn-about-abuse/why-its-so-difficult-to-leave.
2. Kim Saeed, "Long-Term Narcissistic Abuse Can Cause Brain Damage," Psych Central (blog), October 20, 2017, https://psychcentral.com/blog/liberation/2017/10/long-term-narcissistic-abuse-can-cause-brain-damage.
3. Daniel Goleman, "Social Intelligence: The New Science of Human Relationships" (New York: Bantam, 2006).
4. Daniel Goleman and Richard E. Boyatzis, "Social Intelligence and the Biology of Leadership," *Harvard Business Review*, September 2008, https://hbr.org/2008/09/social-intelligence-and-the-biology-of-leadership.

5. Saeed, "Long-Term Narcissistic Abuse."
6. Goleman and Boyatzis, "Social Intelligence and the Biology of Leadership."
7. Bessel van der Kolk, *The Body Keeps the Score: Brain, Mind, and Body in the Healing of Trauma* (New York: Viking, 2014).
8. Francine Shapiro, "The Role of Eye Movement Desensitization and Reprocessing (EMDR) Therapy in Medicine: Addressing the Psychological and Physical Symptoms Stemming from Adverse Life Experiences," *Permanente Journal* 18, no. 1 (Winter 2014): 71–77, https://www.ncbi.nlm.nih.gov/pmc/articles/PMC3951033.
9. Andrew P. Smith, "Chewing Gum and Stress Reduction," *Journal of Clinical and Translational Research* 2, no. 2 (June 2016): 51–52, https://www.ncbi.nlm.nih.gov/pmc/articles/PMC6410656.

CHAPTER 7: WHY WE FALL FOR THE NARCISSIST

1. Linda C. Gallo, Wendy M. Troxel, Karen A. Matthews, et al., "Marital Status and Quality in Middle-Aged Women: Associations with Levels and Trajectories of Cardiovascular Risk Factors," *Health Psychology* 22, no. 5 (September 2003): 453–463, https://pubmed.ncbi.nlm.nih.gov/14570528/.
2. Harvard Health Publishing, "Strengthen Relationships for Longer, Healthier Life," January 18, 2011, https://www.health.harvard.edu/healthbeat/strengthen-relationships-for-longer-healthier-life.
3. Peg Streep, "Why We Fall for Narcissists," *Psychology Today* (blog), June 4, 2014, https://www.psychologytoday.com/us/blog/tech-support/201406/why-we-fall-narcissists.
4. Streep, "Why We Fall for Narcissists."

CHAPTER 8: "WHAT A COINCIDENCE!"—THE LURING PHASE

1. Emily A. Vogels, "The State of Online Harassment," Pew Research Center, January 13, 2021, https://www.pewresearch.org/internet/2021/01/13/the-state-of-online-harassment/.

CHAPTER 9: "WE'RE SOULMATES!"—THE LOVE-BOMBING PHASE

1. Margaret Thaler Singer, with Janja Lalich, *Cults in Our Midst: The Continuing Fight Against Their Hidden Threat* (Hoboken, NJ: Jossey-Bass, 1969).
2. Encyclopedia MDPI, "Love Bombing," 2022, https://encyclopedia.pub/entry/30452.

3. Cleveland Clinic, "What Is Love Bombing?" January 31, 2023, https://health.clevelandclinic.org/love-bombing.
4. Elijah Akin, "What Comes After Love Bombing with a Narcissist?" October 7, 2023, https://unfilteredd.net/what-comes-after-love-bombing-with-a-narcissist/.

CHAPTER 11: "KICKED TO THE CURB"—THE DISCARD PHASE
1. Harvard Medical School, "Love and the Brain," https://hms.harvard.edu/news-events/publications-archive/brain/love-brain.
2. Laura Lambert, "Stockholm Syndrome," April 27, 2018, https://law.syracuse.edu/wp-content/uploads/ARTICLE_2_Attached_to_Pander_Report.pdf.
3. Ena Dahl, "Trauma Bonding Is the Drug That Makes Abuse Feel Like Love," February 26, 2020, https://medium.com/dont-believe-a-word-she-says/trauma-bonding-is-the-drug-that-makes-abuse-feel-like-love-c9987cbc9f13.

CHAPTER 13: TRAUMA BONDING, GUILT, AND SHAME: THE CYCLE OF ABUSE
1. Andrew P. Morrison, The Culture of Shame (New York: Ballantine Books, 1996).

CHAPTER 14: WHY WE STAY: THE TRAUMA BOND
1. Harvard Medical School, "Love and the Brain," https://hms.harvard.edu/news-events/publications-archive/brain/love-brain.
2. Harvard Medical School, "Love and the Brain."
3. Ena Dahl, "Trauma Bonding Is the Drug That Makes Abuse Feel Like Love," February 26, 2020, https://medium.com/dont-believe-a-word-she-says/trauma-bonding-is-the-drug-that-makes-abuse-feel-like-love-c9987cbc9f13.
4. Laura Lambert, "Stockholm Syndrome," April 27, 2018, https://law.syracuse.edu/wp-content/uploads/ARTICLE_2_Attached_to_Pander_Report.pdf.
5. Psyche Central, "Anxious Attachment Style: Signs, Causes, and How to Change," June 22, 2022, https://psychcentral.com/health/anxious-attachment-style-signs.
6. Psyche Central, "Anxious Attachment Style."

7. Anna Drescher, "Avoidant Attachment Style: Causes, Signs, Triggers & How to Heal," Simply Psychology, January 23, 2024, https://www.simplypsychology.org/avoidant-attachment-style.
8. Silvi Saxena, "Disorganized Attachment: Definitions, Causes & Signs," Choosing Therapy, October 19, 2022, https://www.choosingtherapy.com/disorganized-attachment/.
9. Christopher Guider, "Creating Secure Attachment," https://www.therapistaid.com/therapy-article/creating-secure-attachment.

CHAPTER 15: "I BELIEVE YOU!"—DOMESTIC VIOLENCE

1. Tina Swithin, "Reunification Camps and the Alienation Industry," One Mom's Battle (blog), https://www.onemomsbattle.com/blog/reunification-camps-and-the-alienation-industry.
2. Center for Judicial Excellence, "Forced "Reunification Camps," 2022, https://centerforjudicialexcellence.org/reunificationcamps.
3. Jackie Davis, Cabot Police Department, April 2014, https://www.cji.edu/wp-content/uploads/2019/04/domestic_abuse_report.pdf/.
4. Very Well Mind, "9 Reasons the Cycle of Abuse Continues," https://www.verywellmind.com/the-cycle-of-sexual-abuse-22460.
5. Domestic Abuse Bill 2020, https://www.gov.uk/government/publications/domestic-abuse-bill-2020-factsheets/domestic-abuse-bill-2020-overarching-factsheet.
6. Conor Friedersdorf, "Police Have a Much Bigger Domestic-Abuse Problem Than the NFL Does," *The Atlantic*, September 19, 2014, https://www.theatlantic.com/national/archive/2014/09/police-officers-who-hit-their-wives-or-girlfriends/380329/.
7. Patricia Kime, "Pentagon Needs Better Data on Domestic Abuse in the Military Community, Audit Finds," May 17, 2021, https://www.military.com/daily-news/2021/05/17/pentagon-needs-better-data-domestic-abuse-military-community-audit-finds.html.
8. Jennifer Shore, "The Role of Patriarchy in Domestic Violence," Focus for Health, October 2, 2019, https://www.focusforhealth.org/the-role-of-patriarchy-in-domestic-violence/.
9. Natalie Pattillo, "For Abuse Survivors, Custody Remains a Means by Which Their Abusers Can Retain Control," *Pacific Standard*, March 29, 2018, https://psmag.com/social-justice/abuse-survivors-custody-battl.
10. Matt Apuzzo, Sheri Fink, and James Risen, "How U.S. Torture Left a Legacy of Damaged Minds," *New York Times*, October 8, 2016, https://

www.nytimes.com/2016/10/09/world/cia-torture-guantanamo-bay
.html.

11. Centers for Disease Control and Prevention, "Intimate Partner Violence,"
https://www.cdc.gov/violenceprevention/featuredtopics/intimate
-partner-violence.

12. Nancy Glass, Kathryn Laughon, Jacqueline Campbell, et al., "Non-fatal
Strangulation Is an Important Risk Factor for Homicide of Women,"
Journal of Emergency Medicine 35, no. 3 (October 2008): 329–335, https:
//www.ncbi.nlm.nih.gov/pmc/articles/PMC2573025/.

13. Associated Press, "Gabby Petito Was Strangled 3 to 4 Weeks Before Her
Body Was Found in Wyoming," October 12, 2021, https://www.npr.org
/2021/10/12/1045344198/gabby-petito-was-strangled.

14. Ending Violence Association of BC, "Non-fatal Strangulation," April 2019,
https://endingviolence.org/wp-content/uploads/2022/07/EVA-Notes
-Non-Fatal-Strangulation.pdf.

15. Heather Douglas and Robin Fitzgerald, "Proving Non-fatal Strangulation in Family Violence Cases: A Case Study on the Criminalisation
of Family Violence," *International Journal of Evidence & Proof* 25, no. 4
(September 2021), https://journals.sagepub.com/doi/full/10.1177/136
57127211036175.

16. Sara Vehling, "Why Strangulation in Domestic Violence Is a Huge Red
Flag," Naples Shelter, https://naplesshelter.org/strangulation/.

17. Hazzard Law Firm, "What Legal Steps Should You Take in Alabama
when Facing Domestic Violence Charges?" https://www.hazzardfirm
.com/latest-news/what-legal-steps-should-you-take-in-alabama-when
-facing-domestic-violence-charges.

18. Shelley Flannery, "Do Women Get as Much Compassion as Animals?" December 30, 2020, https://www.domesticshelters.org/articles
/ending-domestic-violence/do-women-get-as-much-compassion-as
-animals.

19. Mindfulness.com, "Name It to Tame It: Label Your Emotions to Overcome
Negative Thoughts," https://mindfulness.com/mindful-living/name-it-to
-tame-it.

20. Mindfulness.com, "Name It to Tame It."

CHAPTER 16: "RUN LIKE HELL"—CREATING AN EXIT STRATEGY

1. Rebekah Sosa, "Maslow's Hierarchy of Needs," October 24, 2017, https:
//medium.com/re-write/maslows-hierarchy-of-needs-9ead9a46cb14.

CHAPTER 17: HEALING

1. Parkview Health, "Six Tips for Gaining and Maintaining Friends" (blog), October 26, 2023, https://www.parkview.com/blog/six-tips-for-gaining -and-maintaining-friends.

Resources

WEBSITES

Tellatherapist.net. This is my practice; please check out my site for more information.

Thehotline.org. This is a national domestic violence hotline. Note that a security alert will pop up and offer a contact: *If you're concerned your internet usage might be monitored, call us at 800.799.SAFE (7233).* It will also prompt you to clear your browser history after visiting this website.
Text 88788
Call 1.800.799.SAFE (7233); TTY: 1.800.787.3224

https://victimconnect.org/. The VictimConnect Resource Center is a referral helpline where crime victims can learn about their rights and options confidentially and compassionately.
Call or text directly at 1-855-4VICTIM (855-484-2846) or chat online.

TELL A THERAPIST, INC.:

This is my non-profit that will connect you with a narcissist-savvy clinician in your respective state.

HOW TO FIND A DV ADVOCATE:

Thehotline.org
WomensLaw.org

HOW TO GET A RESTRAINING ORDER:

WomensLaw.org

OTHER ORGANIZATIONS:
https://www.domesticshelters.org/
https://www.militaryonesource.mil/
https://www.militaryonesource.mil/resources/tools/domestic
-abuse-victim-advocate-locator/

DOMESTIC VIOLENCE AND HOUSING:
https://www.womenslaw.org is a good resource
In New York, check out https://www.nolo.com/legal-encyclopedia
/tenants-right-break-rental-lease-new-york.html.

BOOKS
Arabi, Shahida. *Becoming the Narcissist's Nightmare: How to Devalue and Discard the Narcissist While Supplying Yourself.* Self-pub., 2016.

Bancroft, Lundy. *Why Does He Do That?: Inside the Minds of Angry and Controlling Men.* New York: Putnam, 2002.

Brown, Brené. *I Thought It Was Just Me (but it isn't): Telling the Truth About Perfectionism, Inadequacy, and Power.* New York: Penguin Gotham, 2007.

Brown, Sandra, with Jennifer R. Young. *Women Who Love Psychopaths: Inside the Relationships That Harm with Psychopaths, Sociopaths, and Narcissists,* 3rd ed. Self-pub., 2018.

Durvasula, Ramani. *"Don't You Know Who I Am?": How to Stay Sane in an Era of Narcissism, Entitlement, and Incivility.* Brentwood, TN: Post Hill Press, 2019.

———. *It's Not You: Identifying and Healing from Narcissistic People.* New York: The Open Field, 2024.

———. *Should I Stay or Should I Go?: Surviving a Relationship with a Narcissist.* Brentwood, TN: Post Hill Press, 2015.

Freyd, Jennifer. *Blind to Betrayal: Why We Fool Ourselves We Aren't Being Fooled.* Milwaukee, WI: Trade Paper Press, 2013.

Hassan, Steven. *Combating Cult Mind Control.* Newton, MA: Freedom of Mind Press, 2015.

Lalich, Janja. *Take Back Your Life: Recovery from Cults and Abusive Relationships.* Walnut Creek, CA: Lalich Center on Cults & Coercion, 2023.

LaRoche, Kaleah. *Rebirth: Traversing the Dark Night of the Soul.* Self-pub., 2013.

Lewis Herman, Judith. *Truth and Repair: How Trauma Survivors Envision Justice.* New York: Basic Books, 2023.

Macaluso, Nadine. *Run Like Hell: A Therapist's Guide to Recognizing, Escaping, and Healing from Trauma Bonds.* Austin, TX: Greenleaf Book Group, 2024.

MacKenzie, Jackson. *Psychopath Free: Recovering from Emotionally Abusive Relationships with Narcissists, Sociopaths, and Other Toxic People.* New York: Berkley, 2015.

Mirza, Debbie. *The Covert Passive Aggressive Narcissist: Recognizing the Traits and Finding Healing After Hidden Emotional and Psychological Abuse.* Self-pub., Debbie Mirza Coaching, 2017.

Morrison, Andrew P. *The Culture of Shame.* New York: Ballantine, 1996.

Ross, Rick Alan. *Cults Inside Out: How People Get In and Can Get Out.* Self-pub., 2014.

Snyder, Rachel Louise. *No Visible Bruises: What We Don't Know About Domestic Violence Can Kill Us.* New York: Bloomsbury, 2019.

Stark, Evan. *Coercive Control: How Men Entrap Women in Personal Life.* New York: Oxford University Press, 2023.

PODCASTS

Navigating Narcissism—Ramani Durvasula
Something Was Wrong—Tiffany Reese

Acknowledgments

If you look closely, the silver linings are in abundance after experiencing narcissistic abuse. It may not always feel like it, but I promise you they are all around us! Make it your intention to seek them out. I would like to thank all of my silver linings:

My family — my brothers and nephew, but especially my son, Anthony.

Yvonne, for always listening to me and making me feel loved.

Natalie, for being there the night I fled and for always being so supportive.

Heidi, Lauren, Paula, Marisa, Jen, Jillian, and Kelly, for also always holding space for me and helping to guide me through so many parts of my own healing, with a special nod to Kelly for being the best literary agent!

Jane, Felicia and the rest of The Red Bank Gang.

My attorney, Doug Anton, for always working so hard to protect me.

Shar, Vinny, Todd, Barri, and Gene, for assisting me with all my wedding dress runs.

Dr. Nadine Macaluso and Dave for being sounding boards.

Gretchen Carlson, for giving me a platform to showcase my run, and Gwen Wunderlich, for seeing the potential in my story and providing me with a platform to be a voice for millions of survivors.

My publishing team at Hachette Go (Renée Sedliar, Nzinga Temu, Amanda Kain, Mary Ann Naples, Michael Barrs, Michelle Aielli, publicist Kindall Gant, production editor Cisca Schreefel, copyeditor Iris Bass) for sharing my advocacy work and supporting me with this book.

Lastly, thank you, reader, for being a warrior in a battle against this sometimes unperceivable enemy.

Index

About the Author

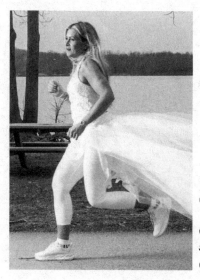

Credit: George Pejoves

Vanessa M. Reiser is a licensed clinical social worker (LCSW), licensed in New York, New Jersey, Massachusetts, and Florida specializing in narcissistic/cult abuse. She is a psychotherapist and the founder of the nonprofit, TellaTherapist.org, as well as a survivor of narcissistic abuse. Vanessa's practice focuses on treating victims and survivors of cults, narcissists, domestic violence, and narcissistic abuse. She is also a long-distance runner and two-time Ironman who is best known for running the state of New York (285 miles in 11 days) in a wedding dress to raise awareness of narcissistic abuse.

Vanessa holds a master of social work (MSW) from the University of Southern California and is also a social media influencer who has been interviewed by prestigious news and media outlets like *People Magazine, New York Times,* Fox News, MSN, and *New York Post.*